RACISM IN PHARMACY

De-Prescribing a Hushed Reality

By

Elsy A. Gomez Campos

Foreword

Structural and systemic racism have existed across all healthcare professions for decades. Pharmacy is an honourable profession, but it is no exception. In a world striving for equality and justice, the issue of racism in healthcare remains a critical challenge that demands our immediate attention. This book sheds light on the systemic biases that permeate our healthcare systems, affecting the quality of care delivered to marginalised communities. It serves not only as a wake-up call but as a comprehensive exploration of the historical and contemporary factors that contribute to inequities in health outcomes. Racism, both overt and subtle, can influence everything from access to services, patient-provider communication, cooperativeness, and adherence to medications and therapies to the very treatment patients receive. This book draws on extensive research, personal narratives, and expert insights to illuminate these disparities and their profound impacts on our education and training, work environment, and how we are represented in our profession and society. It challenges us to confront uncomfortable truths and encourages a dialogue that is essential for fostering understanding and change. As we navigate through these pages, let us remember that the fight against racism in healthcare is not merely a moral imperative; it is a necessity for the health and well-being of all individuals. The insights offered here will empower readers—medical professionals, policymakers, advocates, and especially pharmacy professionals—to recognise and dismantle the barriers that perpetuate discrimination within our systems. May this book inspire action, provoke thought, and ignite a passion for justice as we work together towards a future where healthcare is equitable, compassionate, and accessible for everyone, regardless of race or background.

John E. Clark, PharmD, MS, FASHP Director,

Culture and Climate Associate Professor |

Department of Pharmacotherapeutics & Clinical Research

Taneja College of Pharmacy

University of South Florida

Tampa

Florida 33612

Dedication

"To all pharmacy professionals whose careers have been shaped by the challenges of racism, yet who continue to persevere with strength, resilience, and determination."

"It is sobering to read about the harmful systemic & cultural leadership behaviours in the Pharmacy sector. As a lifelong anti-racism campaigner, it is vital that the sector urgently studies this incredible book, listens deeply to its recommendations and acknowledges how certain institutional practices and power structures are harming marginalised leaders and marginalised folks. Thank you so much, Elsy; we appreciate the work you do and for raising so much awareness".

Abdirahim Hassan (HE/HIM) – Founder of Coffee Afrique

About the Author

Elsy is among the few Afro-Caribbean women pharmacists contributing to the National Health Service (NHS). Born and raised in Cuba, she earned her pharmacy qualifications from the University of Havana. Her pharmacy journey in the UK began in 1996 as a pharmacy technician at a bustling hospital in East London. Driven by her ambition to become a registered pharmacist in her new home, she worked tirelessly to raise funds to pursue her studies at the University of Sunderland, where she completed the Overseas Pharmacists Assessment Programme (OSPAP).

After successfully completing her pharmacist pre-registration training and passing the registration exams, Elsy became a registered pharmacist in the UK in 2001. Since then, she has earned an MSc in Clinical Pharmacy and held various leadership roles across NHS Trusts, working in multiple specialities.

Throughout her time in the NHS, Elsy has both experienced and witnessed racial discrimination within the pharmacy profession and the NHS. These challenges inspired her to become a vocal advocate for Equality, Diversity, and Inclusion (EDI). Drawing on her own experiences of physical, financial, and mental hardship in standing up against discrimination, Elsy transformed adversity into action. In 2018, she founded the UK Black Pharmacists Association (UKBPA), a group dedicated to supporting Black pharmacists, trainee pharmacists, and pharmacy students.

Elsy's activism expanded in February 2020 when she volunteered as a Pharmacists' Defence Association (PDA) Union representative for the South East Regional Committee. By December of that year, she became the first president of the PDA BAME Network, further solidifying her role as a leading voice for change in the profession.

Her contributions extend beyond pharmacy. In 2019, she founded "Romford Speakers," a Toastmasters International-affiliated club that empowers community members to improve their public speaking and leadership skills. This reflects Elsy's passion for uplifting others in all aspects of life.

Elsy's dedication has been widely recognised. In 2020, she was awarded a fellowship from the Royal Pharmaceutical Society, an honour reserved for those who have achieved distinction in their careers. In 2023, she received a fully-funded Roche UK MBA Health scholarship at UCL's Global Business School for Health.

Beyond her professional achievements, Elsy enjoys reading and writing. Her writing sheds light on the challenges faced by Black professionals and pharmacy students in the UK. With this book, Elsy hopes to inspire and inform those genuinely invested in providing equal opportunities to all in the pharmacy profession.

Contents

Abbreviations and Acronyms

TERMS	MEANING
ABPI	Association of the British Pharmaceutical Industry
ACAS	Advisory, Conciliation and Arbitration Service
AIDS	Acquired Immune Deficiency Syndrome
BAME or BME	Black, Asian, and Minority Ethnic or Black and Minority Ethnic
BBC	British Broadcasting Corporation
BPSA	British Pharmaceutical Students' Association
CBT	Cognitive Behavioural Therapy
CDC	Centers for Disease Control and Prevention
COVID-19	Coronavirus Disease identified in 2019
CPPE	Centre for Pharmacy Postgraduate Education
CQC	Care Quality Commission
DPP	Designated Prescribing Practitioner
EEA	European Economic Area
EDI	Equality, Diversity and Inclusion
EMA	European Medicines Agency
ERG	Employee Resource Group
FDA	Food and Drug Administration
FOI	Freedom Of Information
FRPharmS	Fellow of the Royal Pharmaceutical Society
FTP	Fitness To Practice
GMC	General Medical Council
GP	General Practitioner
GPhC	General Pharmaceutical Council
GWAS	Genomic-Wide Association Studies
HESA	Higher Education Statistics Agency
HIV	Human Immunodeficiency Virus
IAPT	Improving Access to Psychological Therapies
ICU	Intensive Care Unit
KPI	Key Performance Indicators
LGBTQ+	Lesbian, Gay, Bisexual, Transgender, Queer (and more)
MPharm	Master of Pharmacy
HbA1c	Glycated haemoglobin (A1c)
MSc	Master of Science
MWRES	Medical Workforce Race Equality Standards
NHS	National Health Service
NHSE	NHS England
NMP	Non-Medical Prescribing
OSPAP	Overseas Pharmacists Assessment Programme
PDA	The Pharmacists' Defence Association
PhD	Doctor of Philosophy

PHS	Public Health Service
POC	People of Colour
PSA	Professional Standards Authority for Health and Social Care
PWRES	Pharmacy Workforce Race Equality Standards
RNOH	Royal National Orthopaedic Hospital
RP	Responsible Pharmacist
RPS	Royal Pharmaceutical Society
SDC	Sickle Cell Disease
SWOT	Strengths, Weaknesses, Opportunities, Threats
TWOS	Threats, Opportunities, Weaknesses and Strengths
U.S.	United States
UK	United Kingdom
UKBPA	UK Black Pharmacist Association
WHO	World Health Organisation
WRES	Workforce Race Equality Standards

Preface

In February 2016, I followed the Trust's internal grievance procedure to raise a series of concerns while working at the Royal National Orthopaedic Hospital (RNOH) NHS Trust. In March 2017, I was dismissed from my position as Deputy Chief Pharmacist. My experience mirrors many troubling patterns described in the Francis Report, officially known as the "Report of the Mid Staffordshire NHS Foundation Trust Public Inquiry"[1]. The report shed light on significant issues regarding staff grievances within the NHS, revealing how Mid Staffordshire NHS Trust employees often felt discouraged from raising concerns about patient safety, working conditions, or management practices. It identified a pervasive culture of fear and intimidation, where those who did speak out were frequently ignored, marginalised, or even retaliated against. Poor leadership, ineffective management, and a lack of transparency fostered an environment where staff grievances were suppressed, ultimately compromising the quality of care and allowing harmful practices to continue. The Francis Report underscored the need for cultural reform within the NHS, advocating for openness, support for whistleblowers, and mechanisms that would allow staff to raise concerns without fear of repercussion.

As a practising pharmacist in the NHS for nearly 20 years at the time of my dismissal, I had always felt a strong sense of safety and professional identity in my role. However, my experience at the RNOH shattered that confidence, exposing a reality I had never anticipated. What's been even more sobering is that, over the years since my dismissal, I have encountered other pharmacists whose experiences bear striking similarities to mine, suggesting that what happened to me while practising a profession I love may not be as isolated as I once believed.

The fact is that the NHS, like many institutions, has deep-rooted structural inequalities that disproportionately affect Black, Asian, and Minority Ethnic (BAME) individuals. These include inequalities in recruitment, pay, career progression, and access to opportunities. These issues often arise from systemic biases embedded in organisational practices that continue to persist despite efforts to promote diversity and inclusion. One day, I hope the issue of racism within the NHS and its impact will receive the level of scrutiny it deserves, potentially through a formal public inquiry. The consequences of this issue can be seen in its effects on individuals' careers, well-being, and health outcomes. Until then, I will focus on sharing my own experiences and those of others I have encountered throughout my journey in the NHS.

In "Racism in Pharmacy: Deprescribing a Hushed Reality," I focus on the systemic issue of racism within the pharmacy profession. The book traces racism's historical roots, examining its continued influence on modern practice and highlighting the ongoing challenges faced by pharmacy professionals.

Drawing from nearly three decades of experience working as a pharmacist in the NHS, I provide a detailed account of the systemic barriers that ethnic minority pharmacy professionals face throughout their careers, from their education and training to their workplace environments. These barriers include unequal access to mentorship, limited opportunities for career progression, and the pervasive presence of microaggressions and overt discrimination. Through real-life stories and the scarce data available, I aim to provide a vivid portrayal of the challenges ethnic minority pharmacy professionals in the UK encounter while examining the broader implications for the profession.

Introduction

Overview of racism in healthcare

Racism occurs when certain groups, often minorities, are marginalised and treated unequally across various institutions, including healthcare, resulting in negative impacts on living conditions, daily life, access to care, and overall health outcomes. It is a persistent issue that worsens healthcare disparities in areas such as mental health, diabetes care, vaccinations, cancer care, maternal health, cardiology, pain management, and sickle cell care, among other health conditions.

In the UK, the NHS Race and Health Observatory has published reports on ethnic inequalities in mental health services, maternal and neonatal care, genetic testing inclusion, digital access, and workforce experiences. These reports reveal significant health disparities faced by ethnic minorities when accessing and using health services, as well as differing experiences among healthcare workers.

Data shows that ethnic minority groups experience barriers in getting into Improving Access to Psychological Therapies (IAPT) programmes, with fewer self-referrals and General Practitioner (GP) referrals than White British individuals. They are also less likely to receive Cognitive Behavioural Therapy (CBT) for psychosis or attend as many sessions. Non-English-speaking women struggle with inadequate interpreting services, while others face poor communication due to mistrust and cultural insensitivity. Many ethnic minority women experience stereotyping, discrimination, and disrespect in healthcare. Additionally, digital exclusion and mistrust of data use particularly affect older ethnic minority groups[2].

These disparities can lead to significant and wide-reaching consequences. When ethnic minority individuals face barriers to accessing psychological therapies like IAPT or receive fewer referrals and limited treatment options such as CBT, their mental health needs may go untreated or worsen over time. Inadequate interpreting services and culturally insensitive communication can further hinder access to effective care, especially for non-English-speaking women, exacerbating feelings of isolation and mistrust. Stereotyping and discrimination can erode trust in healthcare providers and discourage engagement with services. Digital exclusion and concerns over data privacy, particularly among older ethnic minority groups, may deepen health inequalities by limiting access to online resources and support. Together, these factors contribute to poorer mental health outcomes, reduced quality of care, and widening disparities in overall health and well-being across communities.

NHS staff from ethnic minority backgrounds, especially Black staff, also report racist abuse, with studies frequently focusing on nurses and doctors. However, the inaugural

Pharmacy Workforce Race Equality Standards (PWRES) report, published in 2023, revealed that in 2021, Black pharmacy team members were three times more likely than their White British counterparts to report experiencing discrimination at work within the previous 12 months, specifically from a manager, team leader, or colleagues[3]

Inequalities like those described above are worsened by systemic factors, such as institutional biases and the lack of diversity in leadership roles within healthcare organisations. Ethnic minority voices are often underrepresented in decision-making processes, which perpetuates disparities in care. Training for healthcare professionals on cultural competency, anti-racism, and implicit bias is frequently insufficient, further contributing to the lack of culturally sensitive care. Addressing these issues requires structural change, policy reform, and a commitment to equity in healthcare delivery, alongside a genuine effort to ensure the voices of ethnic minority communities are heard and acted upon in shaping future healthcare practices.

Purpose and scope of the book

While the Pharmacy WRES gave a glimpse into the ethnic disparities within the pharmacy profession in the UK, the report failed to really articulate what racism in pharmacy looks like. Hence, this book aims to explore the systemic barriers non-white pharmacy professionals encounter during their educational paths. It examines the challenges they face in accessing resources, mentorship, and equal opportunities. Throughout their training, these individuals often experience limited support and unequal treatment. In workplace environments, discrimination and bias create additional hurdles for career advancement. The book highlights how these barriers contribute to a lack of diversity in leadership positions. The book aims to advocate for systemic change and promote equity in the pharmacy profession by addressing these issues. The book also explores the significant racial health disparities that disproportionately affect patients from marginalised communities. These disparities are not only a reflection of broader societal inequities but are also intensified by biases within the healthcare system, including the pharmacy profession. I examine how these biases influence patient care, medication access, and treatment outcomes, often resulting in worse health outcomes for minority patients.

Through a critical lens, I highlight the intersection of race, gender, and other identities, demonstrating how overlapping forms of discrimination further exacerbate the challenges faced by individuals in the profession. For instance, women of colour, like me, often experience a unique form of discrimination that combines racial and gender biases, making their experiences distinct from those of their male or white colleagues. This intersectional approach allows for a more nuanced understanding of how discrimination operates within the profession and its impact on different groups.

I also examine the issue of anti-Blackness within Asian and other non-Black communities of colour, an important yet often overlooked aspect of racism in the pharmacy profession. Given the profession's ethnic diversity—48.9% (31,421) of pharmacists and 14.8% (3,811) of pharmacy technicians registered with the General Pharmaceutical Council (GPhC) were from Black, Asian and Minority Ethnic (BAME) backgrounds as of 30th September 2023[4]—understanding how these groups can sometimes contribute to racism within the profession is crucial. This topic of colourism is rarely discussed, but it has a significant and detrimental impact on the experiences of Black professionals. By shedding light on these internal dynamics, I aim to foster a more detailed conversation about racism that goes beyond the traditional Black-White binary, addressing the complexities of prejudice within diverse communities.

Furthermore, the book emphasises the urgent need for cultural competency within the pharmacy profession, stressing the importance of understanding and respecting colleagues' and patients' diverse cultural backgrounds. By fostering cultural competency, pharmacy professionals can provide more equitable care and create more inclusive work environments. I also explore the role of leadership diversity, noting that the underrepresentation of ethnic minority groups in leadership positions within the profession perpetuates the cycle of inequity and limits the potential for meaningful reform.

In addition to diagnosing the problems, this book offers a path forward by advocating for systemic reforms within the pharmacy industry. It calls for policy changes that address the structural inequities perpetuating discrimination and outlines advocacy's role in pushing for these changes. The book also presents actionable and authentic solutions, from promoting diversity in educational programs to adopting inclusive workplace cultures, and emphasises the importance of collective action to achieve equity in the profession.

Ultimately, this book serves as both an educational resource and a call to action for pharmacy professionals, educators, leaders, and policymakers. It challenges the pharmacy profession to confront the deep-seated racism that hinders progress and to work toward dismantling these barriers. By advocating for equity, inclusion, and justice, the book envisions a future where the pharmacy profession is more diverse, inclusive and better equipped to serve the needs of all patients.

References

1. Francis, R., *Report of the Mid Staffordshire NHS Foundation Trust public inquiry: executive summary.* Vol. 947. 2013: The Stationery Office.
2. Kapadia, D., et al., *Ethnic inequalities in healthcare: a rapid evidence review.* 2022.
3. NHSE, *Pharmacy Workforce Race Equality Standard* 2023.

4   GPhC. The GPhC register as of 30 September 2023 - Diversity data tables. 2025 [cited
    2025 20/01/2025]; Available from:
    https://view.officeapps.live.com/op/view.aspx?src=https%3A%2F%2Fassets.pharm
    acyregulation.org%2Ffiles%2F2024-01%2Fgphc-all-register-diversity-data-
    september-2023.docx&wdOrigin=BROWSELINK.

Chapter One: Historical Context of Racism in Healthcare

Origins of racial bias in medical and pharmaceutical practices

The roots of racial bias in medical and pharmaceutical practices lie in historical, social, and scientific factors that have shaped healthcare delivery for different racial and ethnic groups. In the 18th and 19th centuries, pseudoscientific theories like "phrenology" and "eugenics" promoted the false belief that non-white races, especially Black individuals, were biologically inferior. Phrenology claimed that the shape and bumps of the skull determined a person's personality and mental ability. Eugenics beliefs are based on using selective sterilisation and breeding to "improve" the genetic quality of the human population.

Samuel Morton's 1839 book, "*Crania Americana*", analysed skull configurations to support his claim of differing mental capacities among what he identified as "separate species," including white people, Native Americans and African people (Figure 1).

Samuel G Morton *Crania Americana* 1839

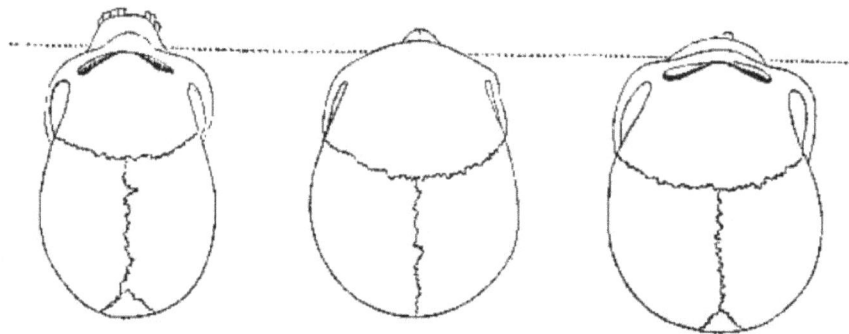

The *first* of these figures represents a Negro head, elongated, and narrow in front, with expanded zygomatic arches, projecting cheek bones, and protruded upper jaw. The *second* is a Caucasian skull, in which those parts are nearly concealed in the more symmetrical outline of the whole head, and especially by the full development of the frontal region. The *third* figure is taken from a Mongol head, in which the orbits and cheek bones are exposed, as in the Negro, and the zygomæ arched and expanded; but the forehead is much broader, the face more retracted, and the whole cranium larger. Having been at much pains to give the *norma verticalis* of the skulls figured in this work, the reader will have ample opportunity to compare for himself. He will see that the American head approaches nearest to the Mongol, yet is not so long, is narrower in front, with a more prominent face and much more contracted zygomæ.

Figure 1: "Crania Americana" by Samuel Morton shows supposed differences between skulls of people of different ethnicities[6].

Morton argued that racial differences were natural and divinely ordained, rejecting the idea that physical variations were shaped by environmental factors. Morton claimed that there were similarities between the skulls of primates and African individuals[5]. Sadly, even today, Black people continue to endure deeply dehumanising acts, including being mocked with monkey noises and gestures. These are painful reminders of the racism that persists both openly and behind closed doors.

These ideas propagated the notion that racial differences in health and behaviour were natural and fixed, reinforcing racial hierarchies. Early medical research often excluded non-white populations or treated them as biologically distinct, leading to generalised assumptions about the health of racial groups.

Stereotypes about race and health continue to influence medical practice today. Misconceptions, such as the belief that Black people have thicker skin or a higher pain threshold, can be traced back to the 1820s and the experiments of Dr. Thomas Hamilton on John Brown, an enslaved man. Medical journals of the time perpetuated racist notions, claiming that Black people had larger sex organs and smaller skulls, labelling them as more promiscuous, less intelligent, and more tolerant to heat and illness[7].

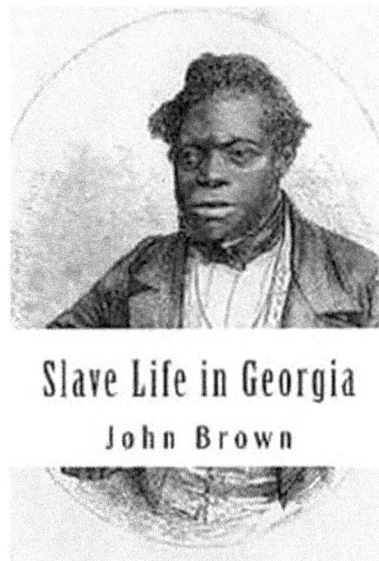

Figure 2: John Brown escaped slavery and published his experiences after he arrived in England.

These harmful misconceptions persist, contributing to inadequate pain management and treatment disparities for conditions such as heart disease and diabetes. Diseases like sickle cell anaemia, which disproportionately affect people of African descent, have been stigmatised and often under-researched. This racialisation of certain conditions has led to insufficient funding and attention for diseases perceived to affect primarily non-white populations.

Throughout history, diseases such as tuberculosis, syphilis, and HIV/AIDS have been disproportionately associated with ethnic minority racial groups, contributing to biased public health interventions and increased stigmatisation of these communities.

In the pharmaceutical industry, clinical trials and drug development have perpetuated ethnic disparities by consistently underrepresenting ethnic minorities[8-10]. This lack of representation results in treatments and medications developed primarily based on data from white participants, which may not be as effective or may have different side effects for non-white populations. When ethnic minorities are underrepresented in clinical trials, regulatory bodies like the Food and Drug Administration (FDA) or the European Medicines Agency (EMA) approve drugs based on data that may not reflect the full spectrum of health responses across ethnic groups, leading to unequal health outcomes. For example, Black patients with hypertension often respond differently to certain blood pressure medications, but clinical research has historically overlooked these differences.

Genomic-wide association Studies (GWAS) have similarly tilted toward participants of European ancestry, leaving other ethnic groups underrepresented. This limits the development of genetic testing and precision medicine for non-European populations, as genetic variants influencing health outcomes in these groups remain understudied[11].

Medical and pharmaceutical textbooks and curricula have traditionally focused on white patients as the "default" standard, with minimal discussion of how diseases manifest differently in non-white people. This lack of representation perpetuates racial bias in diagnosis, treatment, and care[12].

Rare diseases are often underdiagnosed or misdiagnosed in ethnic minority populations due to a lack of diverse genetic data and culturally informed diagnostic frameworks. For example, Fabry disease can be overlooked in individuals of African and Asian descent, as its variable symptoms are often mistaken for more common conditions, such as Rheumatoid Arthritis, for example. Likewise, Hereditary Angioedema can be misdiagnosed as allergies or anxiety, particularly in non-white patients. Neuromyelitis Optica Spectrum Disorder, which is an autoimmune condition more prevalent in Black and Asian populations, is often mistaken for Multiple Sclerosis due to limited clinician awareness. In Addition, Alpha-thalassemia Major, a severe blood disorder that often affects people of Southeast Asian, Middle Eastern, and African heritage, is sometimes missed or misclassified as other types of anaemia. These disparities underscore the urgent need for more inclusive research, broader genetic representation, and culturally competent care in rare disease diagnosis and treatment.

Clinical trials for rare diseases face significant challenges in recruiting participants from ethnic minority groups. Some contributing factors are limited awareness, frequent misdiagnosis, and unequal access to specialist care (Figure 3). All of this reduces the representation of ethnic minority groups in research. Other additional barriers that hinder the participation of these groups in clinical trials are geographic distance, socioeconomic constraints, language differences, and mistrust of medical institutions. Combined with the lack of diverse genetic data, the result is the existing disparities in research and treatment outcomes for underrepresented populations.

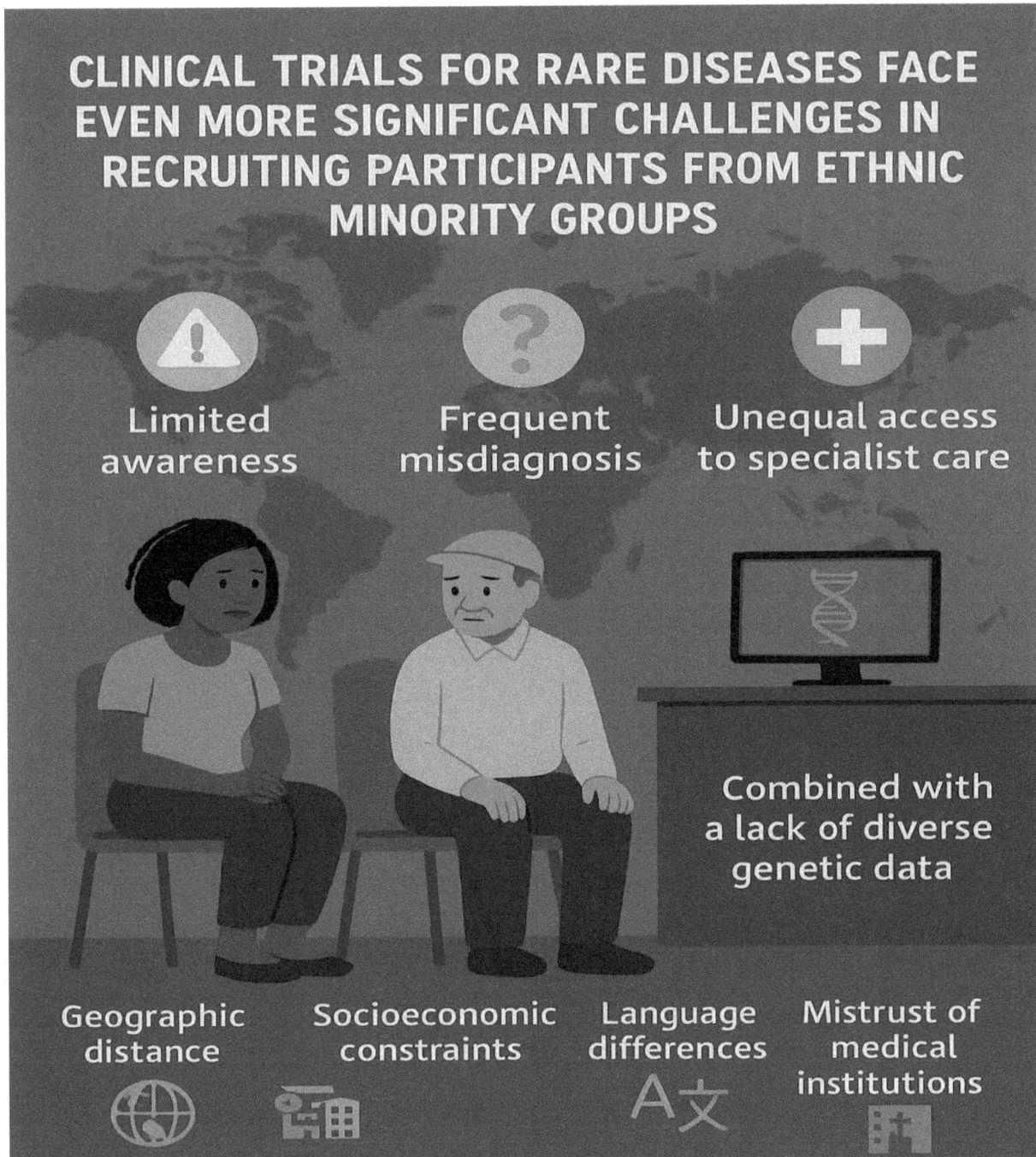

Figure 3: Barriers to Ethnic Minority Participation in Rare Disease Clinical Trials.

The origins of racial bias in medical and pharmaceutical practices are rooted in centuries of scientific racism, exploitation, and structural inequalities. These biases continue to impact healthcare outcomes today, necessitating systemic reforms in medical education, clinical research, and patient care to ensure more equitable treatment for all racial and ethnic groups.

Examples of systemic racism in healthcare systems

There are several notable cases that illustrate the systemic racism embedded in healthcare practices.

The **Tuskegee Study of Untreated Syphilis in the Negro Male**[13], conducted by the U.S. Public Health Service (PHS) and the Centers for Disease Control and Prevention (CDC) from 1932 to 1972, involved nearly 400 African American men with syphilis. The study aimed to observe the progression of untreated syphilis, even though it became treatable with penicillin by 1947. The men were misled about their condition, and the nature of the study promised free medical care, but they were given ineffective treatments instead. Despite penicillin becoming the standard treatment, they were not treated, leading to over 100 deaths. This study remains a symbol of unethical medical experimentation.

Henrietta Lacks, an African American woman, unknowingly became the source of the HeLa cell line, the first immortalised human cell line, pivotal in medical research, as they were the first human cell line that could grow and divide endlessly in a laboratory. In 1951, cells from her cervical cancer tumour were taken without her consent at Johns Hopkins Hospital. These cells, cultured by George Otto Gey, have been used in countless medical advancements. Lacks and her family were not informed or compensated, only learning about the use of her cells in 1975. The use of HeLa cells has since raised ongoing ethical debates about patient rights and consent[14].

Dr James Marion Sims, often called the "father of modern gynaecology," performed numerous experiments on enslaved Black women in the 1840s without anaesthesia under the racist belief that Black women could endure more pain[15]. His surgeries, including those for vesicovaginal fistulas, were conducted without the women's consent. While his work advanced gynaecological practices, it was achieved at the severe and unethical expense and pain of the Black women subjected to his experiments.

In the 20th century, **forced sterilisation programs** disproportionately targeted minority women, including Black, Latina, and Indigenous women, as part of the U.S. eugenics movement[16]. These programs, justified as public health measures, sterilised women without their informed consent, particularly Indigenous women under the care of the Indian Health Service into the 1970s. Black women were specifically targeted based on racist stereotypes of poverty and perceived promiscuity. Doctors often misled women, convincing them the procedures were necessary or reversible.

From 1946 to 1948, the U.S. Public Health Service conducted a **syphilis experiment in Guatemala**, deliberately infecting over 1,300 Guatemalan prisoners, soldiers, and mental health patients with syphilis and other sexually transmitted infections without their consent. The study aimed to test penicillin's efficacy but left many participants untreated. This unethical experiment was not publicly acknowledged until 2010[17].

During the Cold War, the U.S. government conducted **radiation experiments** on marginalised populations, including African Americans, without their knowledge. At the University of Cincinnati in the 1960s and 1970s, Black patients were exposed to high doses of radiation without informed consent. These experiments, framed as cancer treatment research, were conducted without adequate protection for patients and with little communication of the risks involved[18].

In the mid-20th century, many African American women in the southern U.S. were subjected to **unnecessary hysterectomies**, often misled into believing they were undergoing procedures like appendectomies. Known as "Mississippi Appendectomies," these forced sterilisations were part of broader racist policies aimed at controlling the reproduction of ethnic minority populations[19].

These cases reflect the deeply rooted racial biases in healthcare that have led to widespread exploitation and harm of minority populations.

Impact of racial discrimination on health inequalities

Racial discrimination plays a critical role in perpetuating health inequalities by limiting access to quality care, introducing bias into healthcare delivery, and exacerbating social and environmental factors that contribute to poor health outcomes for minority populations.

Racial minorities, particularly in low-income and underserved communities, often live in areas with limited access to healthcare facilities. Many BAME individuals face significant geographic and economic barriers to accessing high-quality care, including fewer healthcare providers, longer wait times, and difficulty finding culturally competent care.

In many ethnic minority communities, mental health conditions are highly stigmatised, and individuals may be reluctant to seek help. Even when they do seek care, they may face additional challenges, such as a lack of mental health professionals who are culturally competent, making it difficult for patients to receive appropriate treatment. This contributes to higher rates of untreated mental health conditions in ethnic minority populations. For example, Black people are more likely to be misdiagnosed or underdiagnosed with mental health conditions, particularly mood disorders and depression. These patients are also less likely to receive evidence-based treatments, such as therapy or medication, compared to their white counterparts[20].

Racial and ethnic minorities experience higher rates of chronic diseases such as diabetes, hypertension, and heart disease. These disparities are driven by both social determinants of health (e.g., lower socioeconomic status, environmental factors, and limited access to healthy food) and discrimination in healthcare settings, which can lead to substandard care.

Minority patients often receive less aggressive treatment for chronic conditions compared to white patients. For example, studies show that Black patients with cardiovascular disease or diabetes are less likely to be prescribed the appropriate medications or referred to specialists, resulting in worse health outcomes[21,22].

In some healthcare systems, minority communities receive less funding and fewer healthcare resources, including fewer primary care providers, specialists, and mental health professionals. These disparities in resource allocation contribute to worse health outcomes for racial and ethnic minorities.

Minority infants, especially those born to Black mothers, are at greater risk of dying in their first year of life due to factors like inadequate prenatal care, poor maternal health, and implicit bias in healthcare delivery[23, 24]. These disparities in maternal and infant health are clear examples of how racial discrimination contributes to unequal health outcomes.

Minority communities are more likely to live in areas with environmental hazards, such as poor air quality, contaminated water, or toxic waste sites. These environmental factors contribute to higher rates of respiratory illnesses, cancers, and other health problems in minority populations.

Lower-income individuals are less likely to afford preventive care, and they may delay treatment for serious conditions due to financial constraints. Education inequality further compounds these challenges, as individuals with lower education levels may struggle to navigate the healthcare system effectively.

Racial discrimination is a source of chronic stress for many ethnic minority individuals, which can lead to long-term physical and mental health issues. This stress, known as "toxic stress," has been linked to an increased risk of heart disease, hypertension, diabetes, and mental health disorders. Prolonged exposure to racial discrimination can also weaken the immune system, making individuals more susceptible to illness.

Experiencing racism and discrimination can lead to feelings of helplessness, anxiety, and depression. These mental health challenges are often compounded by limited access to appropriate care and cultural stigma surrounding mental health in minority communities.

References

5. Poskett, J., *National types: The transatlantic publication and reception of Crania Americana (1839)*. History of Science, 2015. **53**(3): p. 264-295.

6. Morton, S.G. and Combe, G., 1839. Crania Americana; or, a comparative view of the skulls of various aboriginal nations of North and South America, to which is prefixed an essay on the varieties of the human species. Philadelphia: J. Dobson; London: Simpkin, Marshall.

7. Villarosa, L., *Myths about physical racial differences were used to justify slavery—and are still believed by doctors today*. The New York Times, 2019.

8. Fiscella, K., et al., *Inequality in quality: addressing socioeconomic, racial, and ethnic disparities in health care*. Jama, 2000. **283**(19): p. 2579-2584.

9. Murthy, V.H., H.M. Krumholz, and C.P. Gross, *Participation in cancer clinical trials: race-, sex-, and age-based disparities*. Jama, 2004. **291**(22): p. 2720-2726.

10. Health, N.I.o.C. and H. Development, *Health disparities: Bridging the gap*. 2000: The Development.

11. Passmore, S.R., et al., *"My Blood, You Know, My Biology Being out There...": Consent and Participant Control of Biological Samples*. Journal of Empirical Research on Human Research Ethics, 2024. **19**(1-2): p. 3-15.

12. Obuobi, S., M.B. Vela, and B. Callender, *Comics as anti-racist education and advocacy*. The Lancet, 2021. **397**(10285): p. 1615-1617.

13. White, R.M., *Unraveling the Tuskegee study of untreated syphilis*. Archives of Internal Medicine, 2000. **160**(5): p. 585-598.

14. Baptiste, D.L., et al., *Henrietta Lacks and America's dark history of research involving African Americans*. Nursing open, 2022. **9**(5): p. 2236.

15. Cronin, M., *Anarcha, Betsey, Lucy, and the women whose names were not recorded: The legacy of J Marion Sims*. Anaesthesia and Intensive Care, 2020. **48**(3_suppl): p. 6-13.

16. Lawrence, M., *Reproductive rights and state institutions: The forced sterilization of minority women in the United States*. 2014.

17. Spector-Bagdady, K. and P.A. Lombardo, *US Public Health Service STD experiments in Guatemala (1946–1948) and their aftermath*. Ethics & Human Research, 2019. **41**(2): p. 29-34.

18. Moreno, J.D., 2013. *Undue risk: secret state experiments on humans*. Routledge.

19. Saint Jean, A., *Racial Disparities Within Black Maternal Health*. Antiblackness and the Stories of Authentic Allies: Lived Experiences in the Fight Against Institutionalized Racism, 2024: p. 283.

20. Garretson, D.J., *Psychological Misdiagnosis of African Americans*. Journal of Multicultural Counseling & Development, 1993. **21**(2).

21. Fu, Y., et al., *Interventions to tackle health inequalities in cardiovascular risks for socioeconomically disadvantaged populations: a rapid review.* British Medical Bulletin, 2023. **148**(1): p. 22-41.

22. Nazroo, J.Y., et al., *Ethnic inequalities in access to and outcomes of healthcare: analysis of the Health Survey for England.* Journal of Epidemiology & Community Health, 2009. **63**(12): p. 1022-1027.

23. Gadson, A., E. Akpovi, and P.K. Mehta. *Exploring the social determinants of racial/ethnic disparities in prenatal care utilization and maternal outcome.* In *Seminars in perinatology.* 2017. Elsevier.

24. Dreyer, B.P., *The toll of racism on African American mothers and their infants.* JAMA Network Open, 2021. **4**(12): p. e2138828-e2138828.

Chapter Two: Racism in Pharmacy Education and Training

Disparities in access to education and training opportunities

In the UK, data regarding ethnic disparities in access to pharmacy education and training opportunities is notably scarce. This lack of data, however, does not imply an absence of disparities. Rather, it points to a significant gap in research and reporting on the issue within the UK. The absence of such studies could be attributed to various factors, including a general lack of awareness about the extent of these disparities or a limited interest in exploring them. This gap in research highlights an urgent need for more focused attention on how ethnicity impacts access to education and training within the pharmacy profession. Without proper studies, it is challenging to identify specific barriers and develop targeted interventions to ensure equitable opportunities for all individuals, regardless of their ethnic background.

During my tenure as President of the UK Black Pharmacists Association (UKBPA), through ongoing discussions and a genuine interest in the subject, I became acutely aware of the challenges Black pharmacists face in securing places on the Non-Medical Prescribing (NMP) course. Many have struggled to gain access to this critical training opportunity, often encountering systemic barriers. Some pharmacists have even been forced to pay thousands of pounds out of their own pocket to secure both a workplace placement and a Designated Prescribing Practitioner (DPP)—the workplace-based supervisor responsible for supporting them through the experiential learning component of the prescribing course.

This financial burden not only underscores the inequities present but also highlights the lack of institutional support for Black pharmacists seeking to advance their skills. These barriers are not merely logistical but serve to perpetuate disparities within the profession, limiting opportunities for Black pharmacists to fully contribute to patient care as independent prescribers.

Personally, I have experienced being denied training opportunities without any valid reasons, which has significantly impacted my professional development. These obstacles are not only frustrating but also indicative of deeper, systemic issues within the profession. The lack of transparency and fairness in access to training hinders the growth and progression of individuals, particularly those from underrepresented groups, and perpetuates existing inequalities.

Overseas trained pharmacist

Pharmacists who obtained their degrees outside the European Economic Area (EEA) and wish to register to practise in the UK face varying registration pathways depending on their country of origin. Additionally, there are often long waiting lists for the conversion courses required by approved universities. While not all internationally qualified pharmacists are required to undertake these conversion courses, those who must often face significant delays that hinder their ability to practise. My own journey to registration in the UK began with working as a pharmacy assistant and technician, followed by the pre-registration training before I could sit the registration assessment. This process took four years, including the time required to secure funding for the necessary training. Meanwhile, my peers from countries like New Zealand and Australia were able to practise almost immediately upon their arrival in the UK.

In February 2024, in an attempt to address the long waiting periods for the Overseas Pharmacists Assessment Programme (OSPAP), the GPhC proposed a new route for pharmacists from Australia, New Zealand, and Ireland. Under this proposal, these pharmacists would be able to register after a mere three-month induction period, while pharmacists from countries in Africa and Asia would still be required to undergo a more rigorous and lengthy process, including a one-year training programme and an assessment. This highlighted a stark disparity in the treatment of internationally qualified pharmacists, resulting in three different routes to registration: one for EEA pharmacists, one for pharmacists from Australia, New Zealand, and Ireland and another one for pharmacists from Asia and Africa. Under the proposed system, many Brown and Black pharmacists from Africa and Asia would be required to spend significantly more time completing additional studies before being allowed to practise in the UK.

The GPhC justified this proposal by citing similarities in pharmacy education systems between the UK, New Zealand, Australia, and Ireland. However, they offered no evidence to suggest that pharmacists from other countries, particularly in Africa and Asia, were any less competent after completing their home country's pharmacy training. This disparity raised serious concerns about fairness and equality in the registration process.

In August 2024, likely in response to criticism from members of the profession, the GPhC revised its proposal. They announced plans to develop a consultation that would establish a single, unified route to registration for all internationally qualified pharmacists who wish to practise in Great Britain. This new route would reduce the process from two years to one year, combining university study and in-practice training.

The historical disparity in the treatment of internationally qualified pharmacists reflects an institutional unconscious bias towards professionals from certain countries. This is a clear example of why the profession must move beyond historical biases and ensure that all pharmacists, regardless of where they trained, are evaluated on their competence and abilities, not on the location of their degree.

Surely, the most unbiased and fair approach to registering internationally qualified pharmacists is to subject all candidates to the same assessment, regardless of their country of origin.

Implicit biases in the pharmaceutical curriculum

Implicit biases in pharmaceutical curricula refer to the unintentional or subconscious prejudices that are embedded in pharmacy students' training and education. These biases can influence how future pharmacy professionals approach patient care, clinical decision-making, and their interactions with colleagues. Some common examples of implicit biases in pharmaceutical curricula include lack of racial and ethnic representation in case studies, stereotyping of diseases by race, inadequate focus on health disparities, and lack of cultural competency training, including communication with minority or marginalised patients. The lack of racial and ethnic diversity among pharmacy faculty and leadership perpetuates implicit biases in the curriculum.

Pharmacy education often centres around case studies that predominantly feature white patients, leaving students with limited exposure to diverse populations and how to treat the disease in these groups of patients. This lack of representation can reinforce the idea that white patients are the "norm" and marginalise the healthcare needs of ethnic minorities. As a result, pharmacists may be less equipped to recognise or address health disparities that disproportionately affect minority communities.

BlackandBrownSkin[25] is an online platform designed to highlight the clinical signs of diseases on Black and brown skin, addressing a significant gap in medical education and clinical practice. Historically, many medical textbooks and resources have primarily focused on light skin, leaving healthcare professionals less equipped to recognise conditions in patients with darker skin tones. The platform works with "Mind the Gap: A Handbook of Clinical Signs in Black and Brown Skin"[26], a resource developed to educate healthcare professionals on identifying clinical signs in darker skin. Together, these tools aim to improve diagnosis, treatment, and health outcomes for people of colour by fostering more inclusive medical care.

Also, some of the teachings perpetuate the false association of certain diseases with specific racial or ethnic groups. For example, sickle cell anaemia is often taught as a "Black disease," while cystic fibrosis is associated with white populations. While these conditions may have higher prevalence in certain groups, presenting them in this way reinforces racial stereotypes and overlooks the fact that anyone can be affected by these diseases. It can also lead to underdiagnosis of conditions in groups not typically associated with them.

Furthermore, education related to effective communication and interaction with people across cultures is non-existent or often treated as an optional or peripheral subject in pharmacy education. When taught, it is sometimes presented in a superficial way, failing to address the deeper complexities of race, ethnicity, and healthcare inequity. This leaves students underprepared to serve diverse patient populations and address their unique needs.

Addressing implicit bias in pharmacy education will require the integration of bias training throughout the curriculum, including diverse case studies free of stereotyping and representative of real-world examples. Above all, it will require an ethnically diverse faculty and leadership to bring about changes.

Black students and their experience of racism

Undergraduate's low pass rate"

"Subnormal: A British Scandal"[27] by award-winning producer Steve McQueen explores one of the biggest scandals in the history of British education. I couldn't finish watching it when it was first shown on Thursday, 20th of May 2021, at 9 pm. On that day, I went from "100 to 0" within minutes. At 7 pm, I was celebrating virtually the fellowship my peers from the Royal Pharmaceutical Society (RPS) had awarded me and the 180th anniversary of the Society. And at 9 pm, I was sitting in my living room watching the documentary, sinking into a deep depressive state.

The pain and impact that denial of education and denial of a future had on those featured in the documentary was clearly visible in their eyes. It was, personally, too much to bear, so I just went to bed because I was scared. I was lucky enough to attend most of my education in Cuba, where talent is recognised regardless of skin colour. Thinking that your education could be denied because of your ethnicity is scary.

I like to think we have come a long way in the UK; the reality is that we still have a problem. "Is Uni Racist?"[28] a BBC documentary with reporter Linda Adey explores the experience of students who report racist abuse and the response of their university to those complaints. The TV program revealed how the majority of students who experienced racism did not report it. Still, those who reported it usually faced denial of their experience by the university investigation process and an unsafe environment after that.

If we examine the pharmacy registration examination results, it becomes evident that a persistent trend exists: one ethnic group consistently ranks at the bottom of the performance table. This troubling pattern highlights systemic issues, suggesting that universities and employers are failing to adequately support pharmacy pre-registration students from a specific racial background: Black students.

Black students are not less capable, but they have been disproportionately underperforming for years, as the data below demonstrates. This highlights the need for targeted interventions to address these disparities.

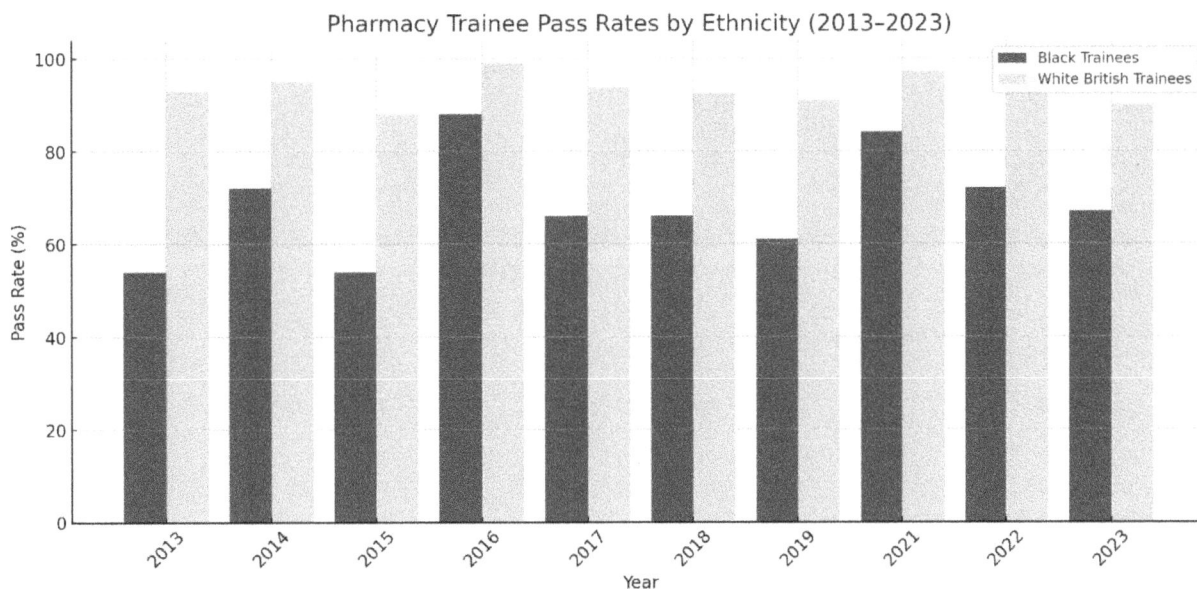

Figure 4: Author-generated figure based on data from the reference number [29].

The ethnicity gap starts in our universities, where Black students experience racism, hardly see any lecturer who looks like them and where academics don't truly understand the challenges many Black students face. Systems that do not recognise nor address the privileges some enjoy and the struggles that others experience are maintained and fuelled year after year.

In February 2016, the GPhC published a report titled "Qualitative Research into Registration Assessment Performance among Black – African Candidates". The report examined the performance of Black-African candidates in the assessments from 2013 to 2015[30].

The report in 2016 highlighted the challenges experienced by overseas students, those with an accent or those whose English is not their first language. Furthermore, it uncovered the sense of isolation experienced by some of the students, some of whom are studying away from family and friends or have family commitments that interfere with fully embracing student life. It is not a secret that some Black students can't fully engage with the course when they have to work part-time due to financial pressures. We are fully aware, since the publication of the report in 2016, nearly ten years ago, that this group of students struggle to get into the pre-registration placement of their choice sometimes because of their background, accent or visa status.

We have substantial data and qualitative evidence highlighting the challenges Black students face within the pharmacy education system. Despite this, progress in addressing these disparities remains limited, and the experience of studying pharmacy continues to fall short of being inclusive and equitable for all. This ongoing gap suggests a lack of sustained commitment to change. The responsibility lies with key stakeholders across the sector, including university leadership, Chief Pharmacists, community pharmacy leaders, and regulatory bodies, who play a critical role in creating and maintaining an environment that actively addresses structural inequities in education and training.

It is deeply concerning that students from Black backgrounds face disproportionately higher failure rates when entering the pharmacy profession. Among the various disparities across ethnic groups, this particular gap highlights a significant area in need of urgent attention. Every single one of these students represents the future of our workforce, and the current situation suggests they are not being adequately supported. If this level of inequality is allowed to persist, it is not surprising that challenges pertinent to equality and inclusion continue to exist within pharmacy practice.

The attainment gap

The differential degree awarding gap (formerly known as the 'attainment gap') and the differential registration attainment gap in the pharmacist foundation training registration assessment highlight significant disparities in educational outcomes. In higher education, the degree awarding gap refers to the difference in the proportion of two student groups achieving a first or second-class degree.

There are substantial gaps for student groups with protected characteristics across many higher education institutions. The registration assessment differential attainment gap refers to the difference in the proportion of two student groups passing the pharmacist registration assessment on their first attempt. According to Higher Education Statistics Agency (HESA) data, an awarding gap exists within the Master of Pharmacy (MPharm) degree program.

In the academic years 2017/2018 and 2018/2019, 91% of white students received first or upper second-class honours, compared to 79% of BAME students. By 2019/2020 and 2020/2021, 94% of white graduates earned a first or upper-second-class degree, while 86% of ethnic minority graduates did, narrowing the gap to 8%. However, a 12% degree awarding gap remained for students of Black ethnicity compared to white students in the same period[29].

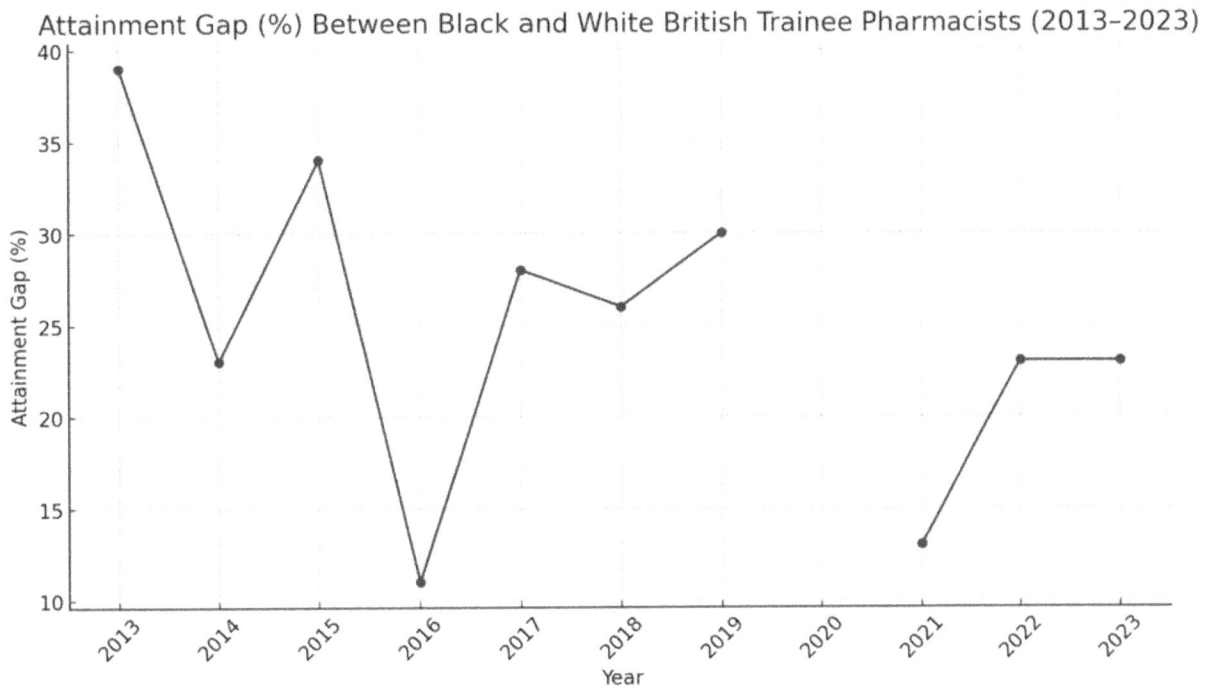

Attainmet Gap (%) Between Black and White British Trainee Pharmacists (2013–2023)

Figure 5: Author-generated figure based on data from the reference number [29].

In 2013, the GPhC reported a 39% variation in the registration assessment pass rate for first-time sitters between Black or Black British: African trainees and White: British trainees. The qualitative evaluation published by the GPhC in 2016 looked into the causes behind this gap. Despite some progress, an attainment gap persists, with data from 2023 showing a 23% gap between Black or Black British: African and White: British trainees in the pharmacist foundation registration assessment for first-time sitters[29].

While improvements have been noted in certain areas, the degree awarding and registration assessment attainment gaps continue, highlighting the need for further action to create lasting change.

The issue of registration assessment differential attainment and degree awarding gaps for Black students and trainees in pharmacy education has persisted for over a decade, and despite being widely recognised, there has been a lack of sustained and strategic efforts to address it. This inaction has potentially had a profound impact on the lives and careers of those affected. Addressing these disparities is not only a moral imperative but also a strategic necessity. Beyond its effect on individual career prospects and opportunities, the profession is missing out on exceptional talent and diverse skills that could significantly enhance patient care, drive progress, and foster innovation.

The reluctance to tackle these disparities reflects a deeply ingrained problem rooted in decades of structural and organisational racism. From the very beginning of their higher education journey to their progression into professional careers, Black pharmacy students and trainees face systemic challenges that have been overlooked for far too long. These inequities have contributed to the lack of visibility and representation of

Black professionals in leadership roles, further exacerbating the lack of diversity within academic faculties and teams. The disparity in training placement opportunities also contributes to these outcomes, as Black students often get less competitive and lower-quality placements. Elevating the overall standard of foundation training will benefit all students and, ultimately, improve the quality of community pharmacy care.

To foster a more inclusive environment, it's crucial to provide training and support for tutors in pharmacy schools and designated supervisors, equipping them to interact with individuals from different cultural backgrounds and respond to their unique needs. Creating a culture that values and respects diversity requires self-awareness about one's own culture and biases. Balancing family commitments with work in the lead-up to the registration assessment has also been identified as a barrier for many Black trainees. Providing dedicated learning time, along with resources, revision materials, and mock assessments, ensures that all trainees are adequately prepared without facing unexpected challenges.

It's vital to continue measuring and analysing performance gaps and understanding where and why they occur. While assessment of performance isn't the root cause of the problem, it serves as a useful indicator. Schools of Pharmacy and the GPhC already collect ethnicity-related data throughout the student journey, but increased transparency and deeper analysis of this data could quickly identify problems that need to be addressed. The GPhC could consider integrating this analysis into the re-accreditation process for pharmacy undergraduate programmes. Additionally, breaking down foundation trainee feedback and satisfaction data by ethnicity, as collected by NHS England Workforce Education and Training, could highlight potential issues related to ethnicity during the foundation training year.

Understanding the wide range of factors that affect a trainee's performance, such as mental health, finances, housing, and immigration status, is critical. Solutions may include providing resilience and leadership training early on to equip students with the tools to handle challenges before they arise. Although various support mechanisms exist for students, it's crucial to ensure that students, particularly those from cultural backgrounds where seeking help may be stigmatised, are aware of these resources and feel empowered to utilise them.

References

25. Mukwende, M. *Black & Brown Skin*. 2020 [cited 2025 20/01/2025]; Available from: https://www.blackandbrownskin.co.uk/.
26. Mukwende, M., *Mind the gap: A clinical handbook of signs and symptoms in black and brown skin.* Wounds UK, 2020. **16**(3): p. 16.
27. Shannon, L., *Subnormal: A British Scandal.* 2021, BBC: UK. Available at: https://www.bbc.co.uk/programmes/m000w81h

28. Webster, D., *Is Uni Racist?*, in *Black & British*. 2021, BBC: UK. Available at: https://www.bbc.co.uk/programmes/p09dhr3f.

29. Doll, A., *Chasing Equality in Pharmacy Training–Closing the Awarding and Attainment Gap for Black Trainees in Pharmacy.* 2024.

30. Johnston, L., G. Cameron, and T. Vanson, *Qualitative research into Registration Assessment performance among Black-African candidates.* Report to the General Pharmaceutical Council.[Online] Accessed, 2016. **31**(01): p. 2018.

Chapter Three: Racism in the Pharmacy Workplace Environment

Implicit bias or racism?

The concept of "implicit bias" was introduced in 1995 by psychologists Mahzarin Banaji and Anthony Greenwald, who highlighted the influence of unconscious associations and judgments on social behaviour[31]. Implicit biases, also called unconscious biases or implicit social cognition, refer to attitudes and stereotypes that people may unknowingly hold. These biases can show up in various contexts, including the criminal justice system, workplaces, schools, and healthcare settings. They often originate from the human tendency to find patterns and make sense of complex issues in the world around us, with culture, media, and upbringing further influencing their development.

Referring to certain acts of racism as implicit bias can sometimes, in my opinion, downplay their severity. While implicit or unconscious bias involves attitudes people may not be aware of, overt and undeniable racism must be called out for what it is. The impact of racism in professional settings is clear from a Chemist and Druggist survey conducted between June 18 and July 27, 2020, which gathered responses from 601 BAME pharmacy professionals[32]. Thomas Cox's "The Huge Differences in Racism in Pharmacy between Ethnicities" is a profoundly poignant read, exposing the stark disparities experienced by various ethnic groups in the pharmacy profession. The survey explained in Cox's article found that more than half (56%) of these respondents experienced racist abuse from colleagues at least once in a six-month period. The highest number of respondents came from Indian (209), African (135), and Pakistani (105) backgrounds, with African respondents reporting the most incidents—78% experienced racism from colleagues over the previous six months. The figure was slightly lower for Pakistani respondents at 61%, and it dropped to 49% for Indian respondents. One Indian respondent noted that the racism they faced often came in the form of "jokes," while a Pakistani respondent recounted being told by a colleague: *"You're OK for a Muslim guy."*

An African participant described colleagues asking "ignorant questions about [my] background," and asserting "'all lives matter' even after Black Lives Matter had been explained [to them]." Another said staff "made gestures behind my back [and] disliked me without cause, despite my kindness... the former manager reinforced the racism those two staff held toward me." A Jewish participant noted receiving "politically charged comments about Israel" from a fellow pharmacist. Disparities between ethnic groups also emerged in those who reported being under "excessive scrutiny" or "treated as intellectually inferior." This was experienced by 46% of African respondents and a quarter of Indian respondents. One Indian respondent said they were denied chances and their expertise was not recognised. "[It's a] constant battle to be respected and acknowledged."

An Arab pharmacy professional described similar treatment, saying: "Despite my skills and regularly outperforming peers, I've been denied advancement." One African respondent stated: "Most locums are BAME simply because they know they won't be treated fairly in managerial roles." Another African participant added: "The psychological abuse I endured [at a pharmacy company] discouraged me from pursuing permanent positions. I turned to locuming in 2019 when my contract ended." One African respondent reported: "At university, a racist student gave me zero on a crucial year-three assessment, which a racist lecturer upheld. Only after I appealed to another lecturer was the mistake corrected, and I earned over 80%." African pharmacists were the most affected by "unjust discipline," reported by 21%, five points above the BAME average. One individual remarked: "Over my 10 years in pharmacy, I've faced disciplinaries over issues that were incredibly minor." Numerous BAME pharmacists reported leaving roles due to racism, ranging from 16% of Indian to 23% of African respondents. Additionally, over 10% of Indian, Pakistani and African participants felt physically or emotionally unsafe at work. One African respondent described experiencing "severe anxiety" as a result of racism. Another said they had "felt unworthy even knowing I am equally capable and intelligent as others"[32].

There is a significant issue within our profession that goes beyond implicit bias. Open racism exists in some practices and remains unaddressed, creating a harsh reality of discrimination that needs to be confronted. Here are examples of intentional racism within the field that are not the result of implicit bias:

1. Ignoring allegations of racism or labelling those who raise complaints as "troublemakers."
2. Blocking career progression, limiting opportunities for acting roles, and restricting access to educational growth.
3. Excluding individuals from meetings, social gatherings, or networking events leading to isolation.
4. Using negative language or making jokes about someone's ethnicity or race.
5. Failing to provide appropriate support or disregarding cultural or religious needs.
6. Relying on harmful stereotypes when interacting with or assessing individuals.
7. Favouring certain employees for mentorship programs or guidance while excluding others based on race or ethnicity.
8. Deliberately failing to share important job-related information or resources that would help certain individuals succeed.
9. Assigning disproportionately difficult or undesirable tasks to individuals based on their race or background.
10. Overlooking individuals' expertise, experience, or qualifications because of racial or ethnic bias while favouring less-qualified counterparts.
11. Publicly questioning or doubting someone's competency or professionalism based on stereotypes, often in front of colleagues or patients.
12. Holding individuals to higher standards or closely scrutinising their work while showing leniency toward others.
13. Minimising or ignoring contributions, dismissing successes, or taking credit for the work of racially marginalised employees.

14. Consistently overlooking deserving employees from underrepresented backgrounds when awarding professional accolades or praise.
15. Inviting diverse employees to participate in public-facing events for optics but not genuinely including them in decision-making.
16. Applying dress codes or appearance policies more strictly to people based on racial or cultural appearance, such as hairstyles or traditional attire.
17. Penalising or retaliating against employees who report discrimination or bring up racial issues, such as through poor evaluations or missed opportunities.
18. Using training materials or examples that reinforce harmful stereotypes about certain racial or ethnic groups.
19. Allowing subtle but harmful remarks or behaviours to go unchecked, creating a hostile environment.
20. Implicitly or explicitly discouraging certain groups from using shared spaces like lunchrooms or lounges.

The Pharmacy Workforce Race Equality Standards (PWRES)

In September 2023, NHS England published the inaugural Pharmacy Workforce Race Equality Standard (PWRES)[3], a milestone following the release of the Medical WRES (MWRES)[33] two years prior and seven months after the latest national NHSE WRES[34]. This pivotal report, rightly acclaimed by leaders in the pharmacy sector, marked a significant step in the profession's journey towards racial equality. It offered a public, data-driven glimpse into the racial dynamics within the NHS pharmacy workforce for the first time.

I could not wait to read the PWRES report. My anticipation was fuelled by my keen interest in the evolution and insights of every WRES report since its initial release in May 2016. I anticipated a document paralleling the comprehensive analysis and detailed information characteristic of the national and medical counterparts. However, my expectations were met with great disappointment. The PWRES, while a commendable start, revealed notable gaps, particularly in its regional reporting across England and in the granularity of ethnicity breakdown.

The MWRES established an exemplary framework, one that the PWRES could have emulated effectively. Table 2 shows the vast difference in the PWRES and the MWRES indicators.

Table 2: PWRES and MWRES Indicators.

INDICATOR	PHARMACY WRES INDICATORS (SEPTEMBER 2023)	MEDICAL WRES INDICATORS (JULY 2021)
ONE	The percentage of Black, Asian, and minority ethnic pharmacists within each Agenda for Change band is 1-9 compared to the percentage of Black, Asian, and minority ethnic pharmacists within the overall pharmacy workforce in 2022.	Percentage of staff by ethnicity in pay bands, which cover all non-medical staff and very senior managers (VSM).
TWO	The percentage of Black, Asian, and minority ethnic pharmacy technicians within each Agenda for Change band is 1-9 compared to the percentage of Black, Asian, and minority ethnic pharmacy technicians within the overall pharmacy technician workforce in 2022.	Relative likelihood of white applicants being appointed from shortlisting compared to that of BME applicants.
THREE	Percentage of pharmacy team members experiencing harassment, bullying or abuse from patients relatives or the public in the last 12 months.	Relative likelihood of BME staff entering the formal disciplinary process, compared to that of white staff entering the formal disciplinary process.
FOUR	Percentage of pharmacy team members experiencing harassment, bullying or abuse from NHS staff in the last 12 months.	Relative likelihood of white staff accessing non-mandatory training and CPD compared to BME staff.
FIVE	A percentage of pharmacy team members believe that their trust provides equal opportunities for career progression or promotion.	Percentage of staff experiencing harassment, bullying, or abuse from patients relatives or the public in the last 12 months.
SIX	Percentage of pharmacy team members who have personally experienced discrimination at work in the last 12 months from a manager, team leader or other colleagues.	Percentage of staff experiencing harassment, bullying or abuse from staff in last 12 months.
SEVEN		Percentage believing that trust provides equal opportunities for career progression or promotion.
EIGHT		In the last 12 months, have you personally experienced discrimination at work from a manager, team leader or other colleagues?
NINE		Staff feeling work engagement: the extent to which staff feel fully engaged in their job.
TEN		Staff feeling 'involved': the extent to which individuals are given (and take) the opportunity to contribute ideas and make changes at work.
ELEVEN		Percentage of BME doctors on royal colleges councils, compared to the BME percentage of the overall workforce

The MWRES was a product of a collaborative effort involving members from esteemed organisations like the Medical Schools Council, the British Medical Association, the General Medical Council, and various Royal Colleges. This coalition was instrumental in crafting a set of WRES indicators that extended beyond the scope of those used in the NHS WRES. The MWRES provided a more comprehensive view by examining aspects such as racial discrimination in medical schools, fitness to practice referrals, representation of BME staff in academic roles, and the attainment gap.

In contrast, the PWRES did not adopt this expansive approach, a decision that I find perplexing. This deviation resulted in significant omissions in the PWRES report. Critical data insights were conspicuously absent, such as those concerning locum staff, academic staff, and processes like referrals and fitness to practice outcomes. These areas are crucial for a holistic understanding of racial equality within the pharmacy workforce. The absence of this data in the PWRES limits our ability to fully grasp and address the underlying issues, hindering progress towards true racial equality in the profession. You cannot help but wonder whether these omissions were intentional.

Despite these limitations, we must work with the information at hand. Recognising areas for enhancement is the first step towards refining future reports. It's crucial to pinpoint specific improvements and strategies effectively to achieve more thorough and insightful reporting in subsequent editions. This proactive approach is key to advancing our understanding and actions in fostering racial equality within the pharmacy sector.

Table 3 gives an overview of the strengths and opportunities evident in the data reported and how we could use them to avoid threats and minimise risks when developing a strategy to tackle racial discrimination in the pharmacy profession.

This SWOT and TWOS analysis highlights the systemic challenges and strategic responses to racial inequalities in the pharmacy profession. Key strengths include an evidence-based, data-driven approach with broad coverage, while weaknesses centre on the underrepresentation of BAME staff in senior roles and higher rates of workplace discrimination. External opportunities lie in developing action plans through NHS trusts and Integrated Care Boards, as well as enhancing education to reduce workplace harassment. However, external threats, such as racial discrimination impacting patient care and staff retention, persist. To address these, the analysis proposes strategies like using data to promote inclusive work environments, implementing targeted training, supporting career progression, and creating robust systems to report and tackle discrimination.

Table 3: SWOT and TWOS analysis of the PWRES.

	EXTERNAL OPPORTUNITIES (O) 1. Development of Action Plans for Improvement for NHS trusts and Integrated Care Boards (ICBs) to address inequalities, offering a clear path for improvement. 2. Improve education and training to eliminate conditions that foster workplace harassment and discrimination.	EXTERNAL THREATS (T) 1. The racial discrimination faced by pharmacy staff can adversely affect patient care and overall healthcare outcomes. 2. The racial inequalities could affect staff morale, resulting in difficulty retaining skilled pharmacy professionals from diverse backgrounds.
INTERNAL STRENGTHS (S) 1. Evidence-Based Approach 2. Data from various sources 3. Comprehensive Coverage	SO STRATEGIES (Use Strengths to Seize Opportunities) 1. Use Data-Driven Approach to produce plans to address racial inequalities and improve career progression opportunities for BAME staff. 2. Develop targeted training and awareness programs that address workplace discrimination.	ST STRATEGIES (Use Strengths to minimise Threats) 1. Use the data to mitigate the impact on patient care by improving and promoting a more inclusive work environment. 2. Develop policies and initiatives that improve the work environment, staff morale, and retention.
INTERNAL WEAKNESSES (W) 1. Underrepresentation of BAME pharmacy staff in higher Agenda for Change (AfC) bandings indicates an inequality in career advancement opportunities. 2. BAME pharmacy staff experience more harassment, bullying, abuse, and discrimination compared to their white counterparts.	WO STRATEGIES (Overcome Weaknesses to Seize Opportunities) 1. Tackle discrimination proactively in the recruitment process to improve the career progression of BAME staff. 2. Develop a support system to report and address racial discrimination.	WT STRATEGIES (Minimise Weaknesses to Avoid Threats) 1. Develop pragmatic interventions to address the disparities in staff experience, such as discrimination and lack of career progression, that could adversely affect patient care and healthcare outcomes. 2. Implement and monitor strategies to improve the work environment of BAME staff.

The release of the PWRES was a highly anticipated event, yet the final report appeared to fall short of expectations. It is concerning to note that despite the involvement of BAME leaders in drafting the report, it lacked the depth and comprehensiveness required for meaningful scrutiny and progress. The absence of crucial data in areas that significantly impact racial equality suggests a missed opportunity for these leaders to champion change and transparency.

Leadership in such initiatives is responsible for confronting challenging issues head-on and illuminating the path to progress. The reluctance or inability to present data critical to understanding and addressing racial disparities raises questions about the commitment to effecting real change from those BAME leaders involved in producing the report. If future iterations of the PWRES do not improve in terms of depth, transparency, and relevance, it risks perpetuating the status quo, leaving racial discrimination unchallenged in the pharmacy profession. It is imperative that future reports demonstrate a stronger, more courageous approach to ensure the profession advances towards true racial equality.

Racial microaggressions – "Death by a Thousand Cuts"

Microaggressions are subtle, derogatory and harmful behaviours directed at someone or a group of people[35]. The acts can be verbal or non-verbal and conscious or unconscious. Microaggressions come in various forms, with microassaults being the most overt. In cases of microassaults, the individual intentionally engages in harmful behaviour, fully aware that their actions may cause offence, such as using a derogatory term to refer to a person of colour. Microinsults, while more subtle, still have damaging effects on marginalised groups. These can include comments suggesting that someone only obtained their position due to affirmative action, thereby undermining their qualifications. Microinvalidations, on the other hand, dismiss the experiences of marginalised individuals. A common example is denying the existence of prejudice by telling a person of colour they are being "oversensitive" to a racist remark or saying that something was not racially motivated. Each of these forms of microaggressions, though different in tone and delivery, perpetuates harm and invalidates the lived experiences of marginalised people. You know if you have experienced a racial microaggression. Expressions such as *"There is no White Privilege"; "There is only one race, the human race"; "All lives matter"; "I don't see colour"; "You are intimidating"; "You sound white"; "Why is there no a "white history month?"; "You are using the race card"; "I am not a racist because I have black friends"; "You must be good at dancing/running"* are examples of "microassaults", "microinsults" and "microinvalidations".

In pharmacy, racial microaggressions are not uncommon. Minority professionals may be frequently asked if they are "sure" about a prescription or recommendation, even when their expertise and qualifications are evident. Those whose first language is not English might be told, "Your English is so good!", "You don't even have an accent" or asked, "Where are you really from?" These comments, though sometimes framed as compliments, imply that the person doesn't fully belong or that they are perpetually viewed as an outsider. A person of colour working in a pharmacy might be mistaken for a lower-ranking staff member, such as a pharmacy technician or assistant, rather than being recognised as a pharmacist or supervisor. This reflects assumptions about the "typical" appearance of those in leadership or skilled positions. A minority pharmacist might be praised or highlighted solely for being "the first" of their background to achieve a certain position rather than being recognised for their individual qualifications and contributions. This can feel like they are valued more for their identity than their skills.

In pharmacy education, microaggressions can create a campus environment where individuals from marginalised groups may feel unwelcome or question whether they truly belong at the institution.

Racial microaggressions can have a cumulative effect over time, gradually wearing down the mental and emotional resilience of those who experience them. Unlike overt acts of discrimination, microaggressions are often ambiguous and subtle, making them harder to address or even recognise immediately. This subtlety creates a particularly frustrating experience for victims, who may question whether their feelings are valid or if they are overreacting. The uncertainty of how to respond, combined with the frequency of these seemingly small slights, can lead to increased stress, anxiety, and a sense of isolation.

Over time, the cumulative impact of microaggressions can lead to more severe mental health issues, including depression, low self-esteem, and burnout. Victims of microaggressions often internalise these experiences, resulting in feelings of disempowerment and self-blame for not responding more assertively. The emotional toll is frequently exacerbated by a lack of support from those around them, who may dismiss the incidents as trivial or not worth addressing. Ultimately, ongoing exposure to microaggressions undermines a person's sense of belonging and well-being, creating long-term psychological harm that can be just as damaging as more overt forms of discrimination.

The phrase "death by a thousand cuts" is a powerful metaphor for this phenomenon, illustrating how a series of small, seemingly insignificant problems can accumulate over time, leading to significant negative outcomes or failures. This metaphor encapsulates the gradual erosion of mental health and resilience experienced by individuals who face constant microaggressions and subtle forms of discrimination.

While the chronic stress and burden of racism on mental health have been widely documented, the physical effects of stress induced by racism are often overlooked and ignored. These include headaches, neck and shoulder pain, lack of appetite, back pain, a heavy chest, tight muscles and an upset stomach, among other ailments (figure 6). These are conditions that are the result of prolonged exposure to toxic stress and systemic inequality.

If you have experienced racism, it may be helpful to reflect on whether you have also encountered any of these physical symptoms and consider if they could be connected to those experiences. For example, I experienced chronic migraine-type headaches for years, underwent multiple investigations, and was prescribed various treatments, yet the migraines stopped entirely after I left the workplace, where I had experienced discrimination.

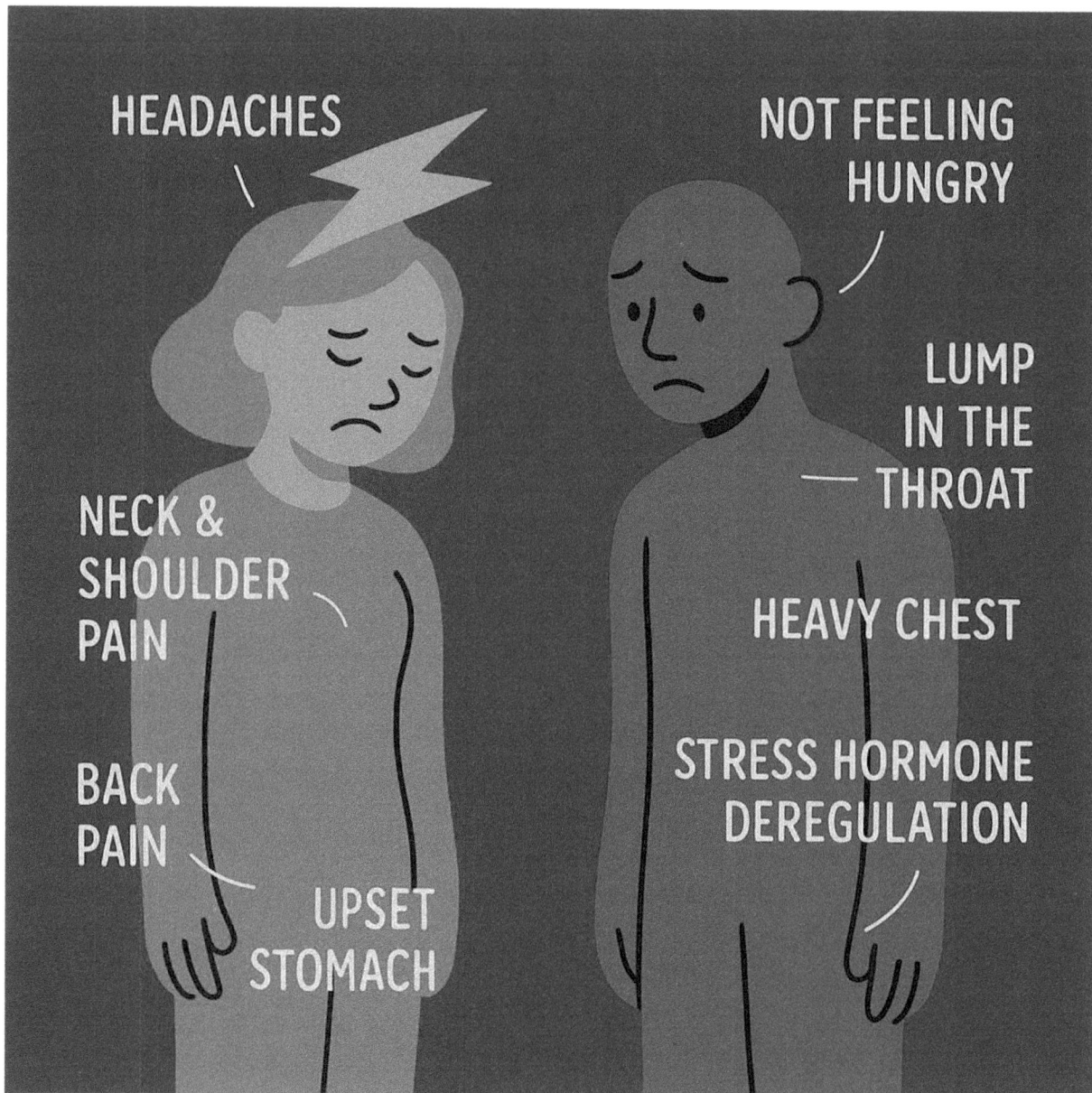

Figure 6: Effects of Stress Caused by Racism.

Chronic exposure to racial discrimination can lead to a range of both physical and mental health conditions (Figure 7). Harvard scholar David R. Williams has extensively studied the social influences on health, enhancing our understanding of the complex interplay between race, socioeconomic status, racism, stress, health behaviours, and religious involvement in shaping both physical and mental health[36].

Racial discrimination leads to poorer sleep, increased inflammation, obesity, and cardiovascular disease, including high blood pressure and coronary heart disease. Psychologically, racism is linked to psychiatric disorders such as depression, anxiety, eating disorders, and psychosis. These health issues demonstrate how the persistent stress induced by racism places individuals at higher risk for serious long-term illnesses[37].

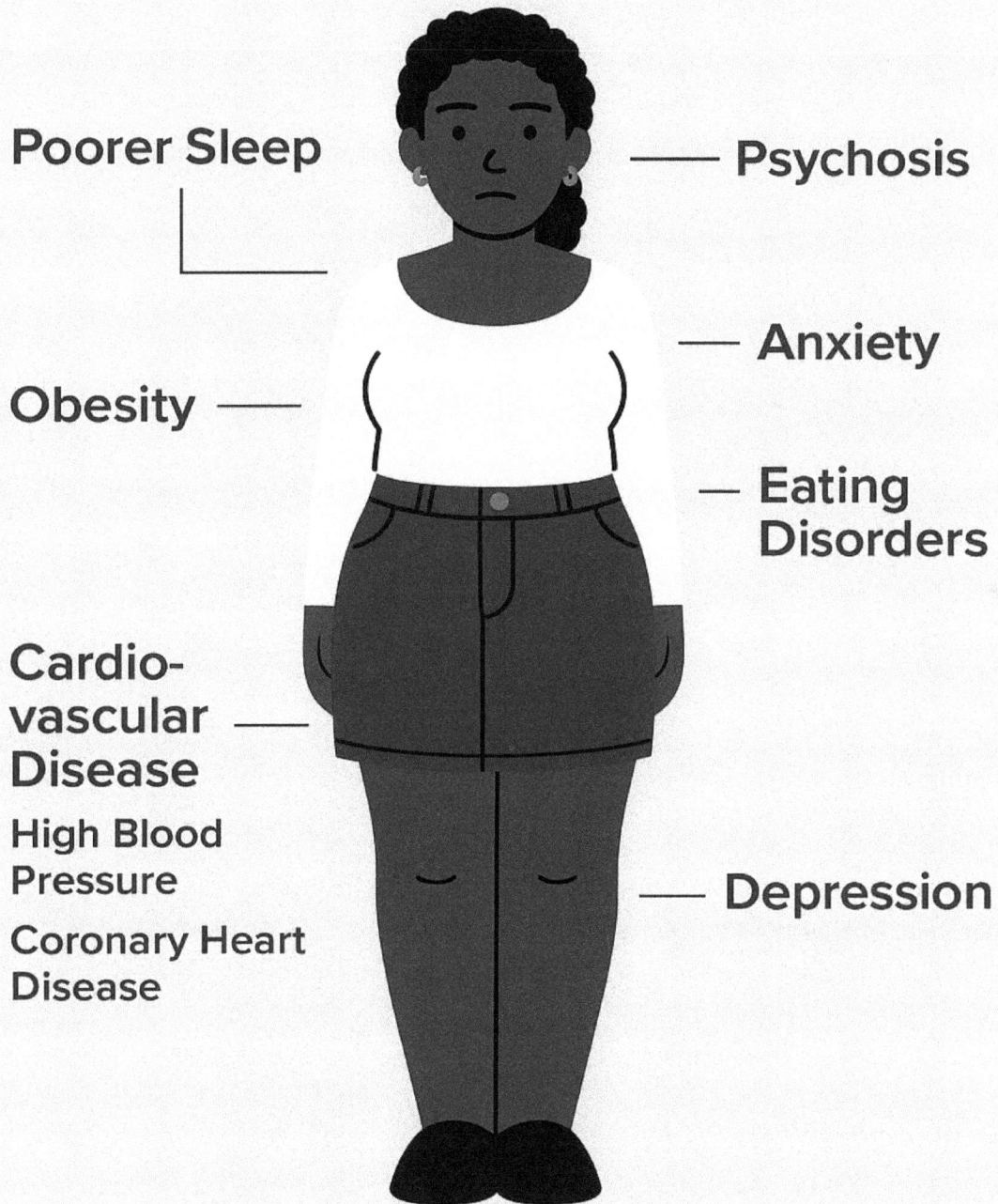

Figure 7: Effects of Racism on Physical and Mental Health.

The health effects of racism go far beyond the individuals directly impacted. They can affect their families as well. When a family member experiences chronic stress, poor sleep, or mental health challenges like depression or anxiety due to racism, it can stress the whole family's well-being and create emotional distress for loved ones. Parents facing these challenges may struggle to provide consistent emotional support, which can affect children's development and sense of security. Financial strain may also arise from missed work, healthcare costs, or limited career advancement linked to systemic discrimination. Additionally, witnessing or experiencing racism can shape children's worldviews, leading to internalised stress about perhaps facing similar discrimination. In essence, racism damages the physical, emotional, and economic well-being of entire family systems, perpetuating cycles of disadvantage across generations.

In the pharmacy profession, racism and microaggressions are unfortunately a reality, often escalating into more overt issues like bullying and collusion. These experiences can further exacerbate the hostile work or study environment, negatively impacting the overall health and well-being of those affected and their families. Addressing these issues is crucial for fostering a more inclusive and supportive environment in the healthcare sector.

A culture of bullying and collusion

The 2023 PWRES report revealed that a higher percentage of BAME pharmacy team members (15.3%) experienced harassment, bullying, or abuse from patients, relatives, or the public in the past 12 months, compared to 12.5% of their white colleagues. Additionally, 25.3% of BAME pharmacy staff reported similar mistreatment from NHS staff, a figure higher than the 21.1% reported by their white counterparts. These troubling disparities have been consistently observed since at least 2015, highlighting ongoing racial inequalities both from the public and within the NHS itself.

Internal collusion is a significant, yet often unspoken, factor contributing to the bullying within the pharmacy profession. Despite its prevalence, many hesitate to acknowledge or address its existence, allowing it to persist as a harsh reality that exacerbates the problem. Though uncomfortable to confront, this issue plays a critical role in perpetuating a toxic environment in our field.

In July 2024, I submitted a blog to the "Chemist and Druggist" to raise awareness about this issue. However, James Halliwell, the Editor-in-Chief, declined to publish it, stating, *"It's a big ask to suggest the industry is riddled with 'collusion' to the detriment of the safety of patients and employees, with only your anecdotal evidence to back that up."* He added that he would not run an article that makes such claims without further investigation or consultation with relevant bodies, such as the GPhC. Mr Halliwell, a business journalist for 15 years, expressed sympathy for my experience while emphasising that he would not suggest the problem was endemic to the profession based on one person's account.

This response reflects a broader unwillingness to confront or even explore uncomfortable truths about our profession. Collusion is a serious issue that perpetuates a toxic culture, harming both patient safety and the well-being of pharmacy professionals. Unfortunately, attempts to highlight this issue are often silenced or ignored, reinforcing the very culture of denial that allows collusion to thrive.

I wish collusion were a problem I had encountered alone. Over the years, I have heard numerous reports from pharmacy colleagues that suggest this may be a systemic issue. Their accounts mirror my own experience and point to a pattern that affects career progression, mental health, and the overall inclusivity of our profession. It's a problem that deserves serious attention, not dismissal if we are to uphold the values of care and integrity that our profession claims to champion.

Collusion occurs when there is a secretive or illegal agreement between two or more parties to deceive, mislead, or defraud others. It often involves working together to achieve a common objective through dishonest or unethical means. Collusion can take various forms in the workplace. In pharmacy, I have witnessed and been told of staff colluding to deflect attention from their poor performance or discrimination towards others.

Sadly, many of the struggles faced by the pharmacy workforce are often acknowledged superficially but fail to result in meaningful change. The practice of barring certain individuals from obtaining jobs (blacklisting) as punishment for speaking up and dysfunctional decision-making (groupthink) that manifests in toxic staff collusion to justify discrimination and poor performance are, in my opinion, commonly denied and overlooked.

Based on my personal experiences and the stories shared with me by peers, I believe that a culture of collusion and groupthink can sometimes emerge in pharmacy environments. These behaviours, while often denied, may contribute to unfair treatment, hinder diversity, and compromise psychological safety for professionals, particularly those from underrepresented backgrounds. Such behaviours persist because there are no meaningful consequences for those responsible for such harmful actions.

Collusion has no place in healthcare because it directly threatens patient safety. It causes me great sadness to hear testimonies from pharmacy professionals driven out of their workplace by it. When staff collude, they may cover up mistakes, ignore protocol breaches or falsify records to protect each other.

This lack of transparency can lead to undetected errors, compromised care standards, and a culture where patient safety is not prioritised. Collusion undermines trust, accountability, and the ability to address issues promptly, increasing the risk of harm to patients and damaging the overall integrity of the healthcare system.

Moreover, collusion can severely damage employee trust, making the workplace unsafe. Knowledge of collusion can demoralise employees who value integrity, decreasing job satisfaction and productivity. It can also lead to the misallocation of resources, favouritism, and inefficiencies, resulting in suboptimal organisational outcomes.

On the other hand, when employees and leaders act with integrity, trust within the team is fostered. Colleagues can rely on each other, knowing everyone will act honestly and consistently. Open and honest communication reduces suspicion and builds a transparent work environment where employees feel informed and valued. In pharmacy, we need all leaders to act with integrity and set a strong example for their teams, reinforcing positive behaviours and ethical standards.

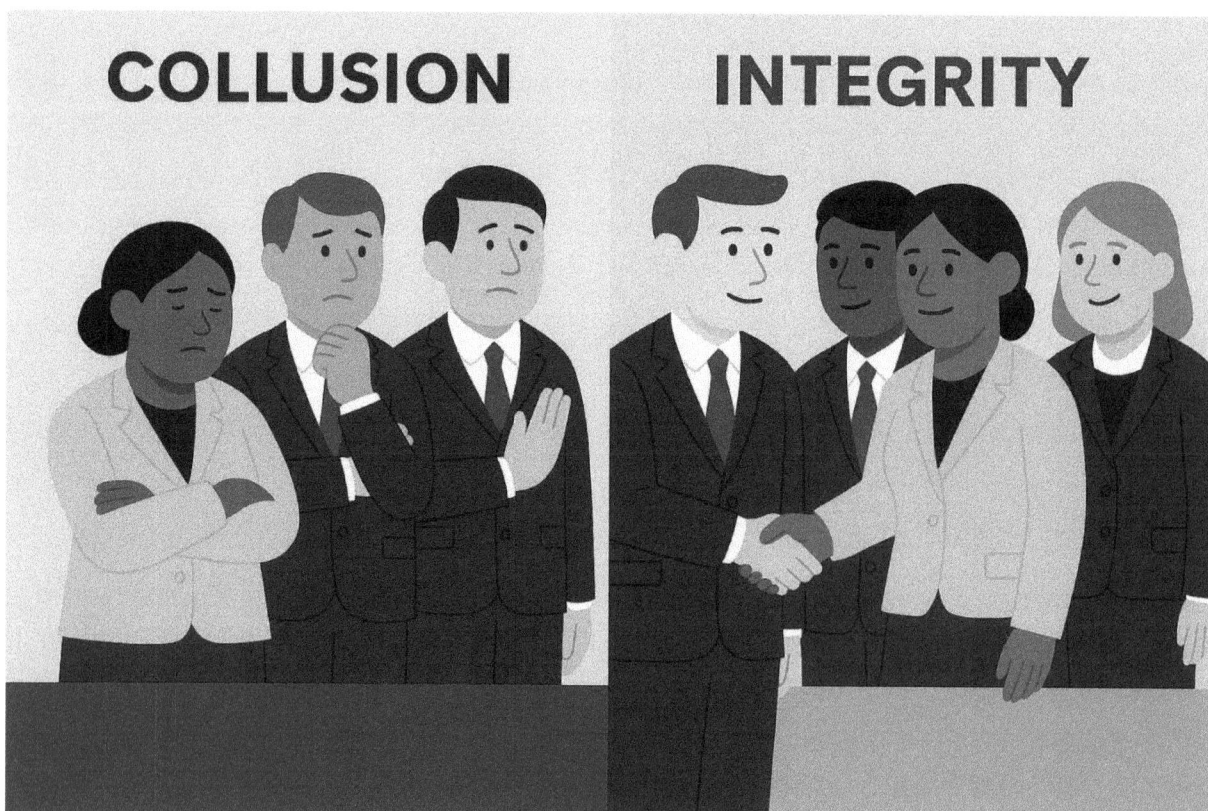

Figure 8: Collusion vs. Integrity: The Impact of Workplace Culture on Trust and Team Dynamics.

The human and financial cost of bullying in the NHS

Bullying and harassment are far from harmless, and they come at a staggering cost. A study published in *Public Money and Management* estimates that these issues cost the

NHS an astonishing £2.3 billion annually[38]. These costs are driven by factors such as staff sickness absence, presenteeism (working while experiencing bullying), high employee turnover, reduced productivity, and compensation claims. However, researchers suggest the actual figure may be even higher, as some costs, such as counselling for staff who witness bullying or the expenses of investigations by regulatory bodies like the Care Quality Commission (CQC), are not fully quantified.

Beyond the financial impact, bullying in the NHS has profound implications for patient care. The study highlights that bullied healthcare workers are less likely to speak out, admit mistakes, or collaborate effectively in team settings. These behaviours compromise patient safety and the quality of care delivered. A culture of bullying erodes staff confidence, impairs their ability to perform their duties, and creates a ripple effect that negatively impacts both colleagues and patients.

The study also emphasised that the NHS's annual staff surveys fail to capture many behaviours linked to bullying. Critical factors such as bystander experiences, workplace incivilities, and employee satisfaction with anti-bullying policies and procedures remain undocumented. This gap parallels challenges seen in the pharmacy profession and highlights the need for better tools and methodologies to measure and address workplace bullying comprehensively.

To tackle bullying, harassment, and collusion effectively, we must implement targeted interventions aimed at improving workplace culture. This includes enhancing support systems, creating environments where employees feel safe to report incidents, and fostering leadership accountability. By addressing these systemic issues, the NHS can significantly reduce the financial and human costs of bullying, fostering a healthier and more productive workplace for its staff and patients alike.

It is essential to recognise that bullying and harassment in the NHS are not just financial burdens; they represent moral and operational failures. Tackling these issues is critical to improving staff well-being, safeguarding patient care, and ensuring the long-term sustainability of the health service.

I hope to see the pharmacy profession take a leading role in driving the implementation of meaningful interventions to eliminate bullying within the NHS. As a diverse and highly visible part of the healthcare workforce in the UK, pharmacy has the potential to set the standard for how a respectful, supportive, and inclusive professional culture should look. We can model how to create environments where staff feel psychologically safe, empowered to speak up, and confident that their concerns will be taken seriously and addressed appropriately. By championing authenticity, transparency, accountability, and compassionate leadership, the pharmacy profession can serve as an example for the wider NHS, demonstrating that tackling bullying is not only possible but essential for both staff wellbeing and patient care.

References

31. Greenwald, A.G. and M.R. Banaji, *Implicit social cognition: attitudes, self-esteem, and stereotypes.* Psychological Review, 1995. **102**(1): p. 4.

32. .Cox, T. The huge differences in racism in pharmacy between ethnicities. 2020; Available at: : https://www.chemistanddruggist.co.uk/CD005219/The-huge-differences-in-racism-in-pharmacy-between-ethnicities.

33. NHSE, *Medical Workforce Race Equality Standard (MWRES) 2020.* 2021. p. 29. Available at: https://www.england.nhs.uk/wp-content/uploads/2021/07/MWRES-DIGITAL-2020_FINAL.pdf.

34. NHSE, *NHS Workforce Race Equality Standard (WRES)2022 data analysis report for NHS trusts.* 2023: NHSE. p. 43. Available at: https://www.england.nhs.uk/long-read/nhs-workforce-race-equality-standard-wres2022-data-analysis-report-for-nhs-trusts/.

35. Sue, D.W. and L. Spanierman, *Microaggressions in everyday life.* 2020: John Wiley & Sons.

36. Williams, D.R., Race, socioeconomic status, and health the added effects of racism and discrimination. Annals of the New York Academy of Sciences, 1999. 896(1): p. 173-188.

37. Medical News Today. (2023). Effects of racism: How racism can affect physical and mental health. [online] Available at: https://www.medicalnewstoday.com/articles/effects-of-racism.

38. Kline, R. and D. Lewis, The price of fear: estimating the financial cost of bullying and harassment to the NHS in England. Public money & management, 2019. 39(3): p. 166-174.

Chapter Four: The Hushed Reality

Experiencing everyday racism in pharmacy.

Everyday racism is the routine, often subtle, form of discrimination that many individuals from minoritised ethnic backgrounds encounter in their professional environments. For pharmacy professionals, these experiences can manifest in numerous ways that, while individually may seem trivial to some, collectively create a hostile and inequitable workplace culture.

One common manifestation, which is easy to carry out in a clinical environment, is the fabrication or exaggeration of performance issues. Pharmacy professionals may find themselves disproportionately scrutinised, with minor mistakes magnified or baseless concerns raised, leading to stalled career progression, missed promotions, or even disciplinary actions not equally applied to others.

Personal appearance and cultural expression often become targets for microaggressions. Comments on clothing choices, such as traditional dress, culturally significant hairstyle or remarks about food brought into the tea room, can reinforce exclusion. Such comments, often framed as jokes or casual observations, subtly undermine a person's professional identity and belonging.

Communication styles are another frequent focus. Pharmacy professionals with diverse accents may face unfair assumptions about their competence or intelligence. Likewise, natural mannerisms, such as expressive use of hands while speaking, can be misinterpreted as aggressive or unprofessional, feeding into harmful stereotypes.

Access to development opportunities often reflects deeper systemic bias. Talented pharmacy professionals may be denied mentoring, training, and leadership development programs, with gatekeeping behaviours rationalised under the guise of "fit", "not necessary for the role", or "readiness." These missed opportunities perpetuate inequality at more senior levels within the profession.

Finally, isolation is a persistent and harmful experience for many. Being the only individual of a particular ethnic background within a team or department can lead to feelings of invisibility, tokenism, or hyper-visibility, where minor actions are disproportionately noticed and criticised. This lack of genuine inclusion impacts the mental health of those affected and inhibits their career growth and job satisfaction.

Everyday racism in pharmacy does not always appear overtly hostile; rather, it is embedded into workplace interactions, feedback, decision-making, and organisational cultures. Addressing it requires a proactive commitment to equity, active allyship, and systemic change to create truly inclusive environments where all pharmacy professionals can thrive.

Experiencing racism as a locum employee

Experiencing racism as a locum pharmacy professional is particularly disheartening, especially in a role already fraught with job insecurity. I am personally aware of at least one Black female locum pharmacist working in a hospital who was unfairly blamed for a clinical error she did not make, leading to the termination of her contract. Such practices are not only deeply troubling but also dangerous, raising serious concerns about the integrity and fairness within our profession. The targeting of individuals based on race in such a critical profession can have far-reaching consequences, impacting patient safety, career progression, and the mental well-being of those involved.

In the NHS, where many locum pharmacy staff are employed, data reveals that Black British bank workers are nearly six times more likely to face formal disciplinary action than their white colleagues. The first NHS Bank WRES report, which includes data on over 171,000 temporary NHS workers, also found that BME temporary workers were 1.4 times more likely to face formal dismissal for conduct or capability issues compared to their white counterparts. Additionally, nearly one-third (27%) of BME workers reported experiencing discrimination from patients, compared to just 7% of white workers. Over 36% of BME staff also reported encountering harassment, bullying, or abuse from patients, in contrast to 31% of white staff[39]. These alarming figures underscore the structural inequalities that Black locum pharmacy professionals frequently encounter. The disproportionate handling of disciplinary actions reflects broader systemic racism, where the competence and professionalism of Black staff are unjustly scrutinised, often without valid cause.

Locum staff, in general, operate under unstable conditions, with contracts that can be terminated on as little as a week's notice, frequently without any clear explanation. This leaves locum staff—particularly those from ethnic minority backgrounds—exposed and vulnerable to discrimination, at the mercy of employers who may harbour implicit or explicit biases. Subtle forms of racism, such as being labelled "not a good fit" or "not liked" by a team, are often masked as professional judgment when, in reality, they stem from racial prejudices. These discriminatory practices can result in contract terminations or poor treatment without formal repercussions for those responsible.

In such situations, locum pharmacy professionals face a difficult dilemma: either endure the mistreatment and hope it remains bearable or leave quietly. The fear of raising a formal complaint is pervasive because doing so could jeopardise future opportunities in a profession where reputation and word-of-mouth connections hold substantial weight. The pharmacy sector, particularly within hospital settings, is often a tightly knit community where "everyone knows everyone," making it nearly impossible for those who experience discrimination to speak out without risking further harm to their careers. This creates a culture of silence, where locum staff who face racism are effectively left without recourse, trapped between their personal dignity and professional survival.

Adding to the complexity, the PWRES does not currently explore the experiences of racism among locum pharmacy staff, a glaring omission given that this group is uniquely vulnerable to unfair treatment. Throughout my pharmacy career, I have witnessed locum pharmacists, especially those from minority backgrounds, being treated differently and, too often, unfairly. Many have had their contracts terminated for reasons as vague as not being "liked" or "not fitting in" with a team, despite their competence and professionalism. These subjective judgments, often marked with racial bias, have a profound impact on the livelihoods and careers of BAME locum staff.

There are many questions that need to be asked and answered to make our profession more inclusive and fair. How many locum pharmacy professionals have had their contracts unjustly terminated for reasons unrelated to their performance? How often do racial biases influence decisions about who stays and who goes? Why is there a lack of transparency and accountability in such situations? Most importantly, why do we, as a profession, shy away from asking these questions in the first place?

The answers to these questions are crucial if we are to dismantle the systemic racism that still affects parts of the pharmacy profession. Until we confront these uncomfortable realities and commit to real, structural changes, the cycle of discrimination will continue, harming both the professionals who dedicate their lives to patient care and the communities that rely on their expertise.

The Boots' Employment Tribunal case

Hearing examples of racial discrimination in the pharmacy profession is rare. Most cases do not come to the public domain because they are either sorted out behind closed doors or victims do not pursue them due to many different factors related to affordability, the stress it may cause or consequences on career progression, among other things. The Boots case is a rare instance of a case going to the employment tribunal. Mr Famojuro, a Boots pharmacist, won a constructive dismissal and harassment case after experiencing race-related discrimination and mishandling of his grievance[40]. As a Nigerian relief pharmacist managing multiple Boots branches, Famojuro faced resistance from two junior colleagues, Ms Daley and Ms Walker, on 18 July 2020 while working in a Wickford, Essex branch. When Daley publicly snapped at him, Famojuro privately asked her to leave, but she claimed he used an aggressive tone. Walker intervened, criticising Famojuro and later threatened to call the police, falsely claiming he was intimidating her. Daley and Walker also contacted their manager, Ms. Munson, who instructed Famojuro to leave and later called him an "utter disgrace."

Following this incident, Famojuro raised a grievance about his treatment, but Boots delayed investigating it until January 2021. The tribunal found that Boots' investigation, led by Mr Barton, was insufficient, failing to assess whether race influenced the treatment Famojuro experienced. Key claims, such as Walker's police threat, were not properly examined, and the grievance manager lacked specific training in handling discrimination complaints.

Famojuro's appeal was ultimately dismissed, prompting his resignation in April 2021 due to the lack of support and prolonged investigation. The tribunal concluded that the behaviour of his colleagues, escalating from dismissive actions to "highly personalised abuse," constituted harassment. While Walker argued her actions were not racially motivated due to having Black friends, the judge dismissed this defence, noting that such associations do not preclude discriminatory actions. The tribunal highlighted the seriousness of reporting a Black man to the police without evidence.

While the tribunal criticised Boots' investigation, it attributed the flaws to inadequate training rather than racial bias. Nonetheless, it ruled that Famojuro was constructively dismissed and harassed due to his race, although his direct race discrimination claim was dismissed.

The Pharmacists' Defence Association (PDA) represented Famojuro through his grievance and tribunal processes. The tribunal's judgment heavily criticised both the pharmacy team and Boots managers, stating that the handling of Famojuro's complaints severely damaged the mutual trust required for employment. PDA's General Secretary, Mark Pitt, emphasised that the company's support for the employees involved forced Famojuro to endure four years of stress and legal proceedings to achieve justice.

The tribunal awarded Famojuro £45,263.11 in damages and £13,357.25 in legal costs to the PDA, totalling £58,620.36. This compensation, decided in a remedy hearing, included loss of earnings, injury to feelings, aggravated damages, and uplift for failing to adhere to the Advisory, Conciliation and Arbitration Service (ACAS) Code. The tribunal's decision and high award underscored its strong disapproval of Boots' handling of the incident and the fact that some company witnesses fabricated evidence during the proceedings.

Learning from the Boot's Employment Tribunal case

The case of Mr. Famojuro vs. Boots highlights several critical lessons for employers, employees, and the pharmacy profession. The case underscores the necessity of having a grievance investigation process that is timely, thorough, and unbiased. Boots' delays and inadequate inquiry into the allegations, compounded by the investigator's lack of training, resulted in reputational damage and financial consequences. Employers should ensure that grievance managers are trained to handle sensitive cases, especially those involving potential discrimination.

The tribunal noted that having Black friends does not preclude someone from acting with bias or discrimination. Unconscious biases can influence behaviour and should be addressed proactively, especially in stressful situations. Employers can help prevent bias through training on recognising and managing unconscious bias, promoting an inclusive work culture.

The PDA played a crucial role in supporting Mr Famojuro through the grievance process and tribunal hearing. This shows the importance of independent support systems and unions for employees facing workplace discrimination and harassment.

The case shows the importance of maintaining professional respect in pharmacy settings. Junior staff must understand the importance of respecting the authority of Responsible Pharmacists (RPs), as insubordination can impact workplace cohesion, patient care, and the pharmacy's operational functionality.

Delays in addressing complaints of discrimination can harm employee trust, morale, and mental health, as seen in Mr. Famojuro's case. Prompt action reflects a commitment to addressing concerns and protecting a positive workplace culture.

This case reveals the importance of impartial investigations, especially when allegations involve race or other protected characteristics. An investigation that fails to account for possible discrimination can lead to a loss of trust and confidence in leadership. The tribunal noted that Boots' actions damaged the essential mutual trust between employer and employee, resulting in constructive dismissal. Employers should strive to uphold fair and transparent practices to foster a workplace where employees feel respected and valued.

Finally, this case demonstrates the financial and reputational impact of failing to address workplace harassment and discrimination effectively. Employers should view these issues as serious risks, taking preventive measures through training, clear policies, and a culture of inclusivity.

In summary, this case illustrates the need for competent, unbiased grievance handling, ongoing bias training, and a commitment to fostering inclusive, respectful workplaces.

Personal Advocacy and the UK Black Pharmacist Association

In 2018, I founded the UK Black Pharmacist Association (UKBPA) and served as its President for five years. The UKBPA was created from a personal commitment to ensure my experience at the RNOH was not others' experience. The UKBPA aimed to amplify the voices and lived experiences of Black pharmacists across the UK, advocating for concrete and lasting change to address racial discrimination within pharmacy. Through the UKBPA, I led efforts to create a platform where Black pharmacists can connect, share, and mobilise for equity, working collaboratively to challenge systemic barriers that impact our profession.

In 2020, I took on a pioneering role as the first President of the PDA BAME Network. During my tenure, we developed the PDA's "Anti-racist Pharmacy Toolkit," an innovative resource aimed at helping pharmacy professionals recognise, address, and actively combat racial bias within their workplaces. The toolkit, informed by research and the input of diverse voices, should provide guidance to pharmacies seeking to foster inclusive and supportive environments for BAME professionals.

To further spark awareness and meaningful dialogue, I have authored numerous blogs and articles that dissect issues of racial discrimination in pharmacy and call for actionable change.

Recognising that advocacy requires challenging established practices, I have actively confronted various organisations on recruitment processes and the treatment of BAME individuals. For example, I submitted a Freedom of Information (FOI) request to the GPhC to investigate the representation of BAME professionals in Fitness to Practice (FTP) proceedings. The findings showed that BAME pharmacists are disproportionately referred to FTP, highlighting a troubling pattern of racial disparity.

I also submitted FOI requests to NHS England (NHSE) to gain insights into the demographics of pharmacy leaders. Disappointingly, NHSE's responses were incomplete and failed to provide meaningful data on ethnicity and gender representation. Similarly, when I asked "Saxton Bampfylde", a recruitment firm contracted by the GPhC, to disclose the ethnicity of the leaders it appointed, they agreed to share the information but never followed through.

Through these efforts, I have also uncovered at least one instance of non-transparent hiring practices that undermine equality. This was the appointment of NHSE's EDI advisor to the Chief Pharmaceutical Officer without an apparent competitive recruitment process.

Throughout my journey, I've strived to remain relentlessly curious and fearless in questioning racial disparities within pharmacy. However, my experience has revealed a pervasive resistance to change within the profession. This reluctance underscores the work still needed to ensure pharmacy truly becomes a field where professionals from all backgrounds are respected, represented, and empowered to thrive. I aim to spark the transformation necessary for a more inclusive and equitable pharmacy profession by continuously challenging the status quo and bringing uncomfortable truths to light.

References

39. Thomas, R. *Nearly one in three temporary Black and ethnic NHS workers suffer physical violence, internal report reveals*. Independent, 2024. Available at: https://www.independent.co.uk/news/health/nhs-workers-racism-violence-b2606989.html.
40. Courts&Tribunals, Mr S Famojuro v Boots Management Services Ltd and Mrs E Walker: 3219822/2020 and 3204945/2021, E.T. Decisions, Editor. 2023: Welcome to GOV.UK.

Chapter Five: Intersectionality: Gender, Race, and Pharmacy

How race intersects with gender, disability, and other Identities in pharmacy

The double or triple burden of discrimination due to the intersection of race with gender, disability, and other identities in the pharmacy profession creates unique layers of barriers to advancement and inclusion. Professionals who have multiple, overlapping identities have to manage the stereotyping that comes with each of those identities. Women of colour, particularly Black women, face both racial and gender bias, leading to what is often called the "double burden" of discrimination.

Non-white pharmacy professionals who also have a disability often face compounded challenges. They may encounter barriers related to accessibility while also dealing with racial discrimination. This can include limited accommodations for their disabilities during training and at work. Their requests for accommodation may be seen as unreasonable due to a lack of understanding or stereotyping. This may lead to these disabled pharmacy professionals being reluctant to advocate for necessary accommodation for fear of being marginalised. A disability may also hinder the ability to secure a job or promotion if employers perceive disabled pharmacy professionals of colour as less productive or capable of carrying out work that requires physical effort due to biased perceptions about race and disability.

Race and socioeconomic status are things that must be considered because pharmacy professionals of colour from lower socioeconomic backgrounds may face additional hurdles in entering the profession, such as fewer resources for education and professional development. These barriers can persist even after entering the workforce, limiting career advancement and access to opportunities. Socioeconomic status can influence how this professionals are treated in the workplace. Those from lower socioeconomic backgrounds may face more significant financial pressures, leading them to accept less desirable roles or working conditions, which can exacerbate disparities in pay and job security. In addition, those with lower socioeconomic status may find it more challenging to pay for postgraduate degrees such as professional doctorates or PhDs.

Pharmacy professionals of colour from the LGBTQ+ community may experience discrimination related to both their race and sexual orientation or gender identity. They may face exclusion in professional settings, with their intersectional identity making it harder to find acceptance or support within the workplace.

Pharmacists of colour who are also religious minorities (such as Muslims, Sikhs, or Jewish individuals) may face religious discrimination in addition to racial bias. This can manifest in being singled out for their appearance (e.g., hijabs, turbans) or religious practices (e.g., prayer breaks) and facing prejudice based on stereotypes linked to their faith.

Challenges faced by women of colour in the pharmacy profession

From stereotyping to a lack of support, women of colour—particularly Black women—face persistent challenges both in society and within the pharmacy profession. In my own experience, I have been misled by the pharmacy staff I managed, and when I held them accountable, I was quickly labelled as the 'angry Black woman.' No matter how polite, respectful, or accommodating I was, the moment I addressed disrespectful behaviour directed towards me, I was perceived as a "troublemaker" or someone "difficult to work with". This type of bias reflects a broader issue: Black women are often expected to be passive or silent to be accepted, and when they assert themselves, they are unfairly judged. Black women, like everyone else, deserve to be treated with respect and for their contributions to be valued and acknowledged equally.

Within the pharmacy profession, implicit biases frequently undermine the success of women of colour. Their competence, authority, and skills are often questioned, leading to their being overlooked for promotions, leadership roles, and key opportunities for advancement. These biases manifest in subtle ways, such as comments about their hairstyles or clothing that imply unprofessionalism or the dismissal of their contributions in meetings. Microaggressions like these create an environment where women of colour are consistently undervalued and marginalised, making it difficult to thrive in their careers. This kind of systemic exclusion fosters a hostile work environment, eroding confidence and hindering professional growth.

A significant issue women of colour—particularly Black women—face in pharmacy is the lack of representation in leadership roles. This absence of role models and mentors compounds feelings of professional isolation and makes it challenging to find pathways for growth and development. The scarcity of Black women in leadership positions perpetuates a system where their talents and potential are consistently undervalued. As Viola Davis powerfully stated in her Emmy Award acceptance speech in 2015, *"The only thing that separates women of colour from anyone else is opportunity."* Opportunities cannot be meaningfully addressed by the token appointment of one or two Black leaders. There must be systemic change that ensures equal opportunities for all women of colour to advance and lead.

Creating a truly inclusive culture within pharmacy goes beyond implementing policies and training sessions. It requires a fundamental shift in how Black women and other women of colour are perceived and valued within the profession. Pharmacy leaders must commit to listening to the voices of underrepresented groups and taking tangible action based on their feedback. Establishing Employee Resource Groups (ERGs) specifically for women of colour can provide a crucial platform for discussing shared experiences, raising concerns, and developing strategies to combat discrimination and bias. These groups should be given the authority to influence institutional policies and help shape the direction of EDI initiatives within the profession.

Above all, there must be accountability at every level of the pharmacy profession. Institutions must establish clear reporting mechanisms for addressing instances of discrimination and bias, ensuring that complaints are taken seriously and dealt with swiftly and effectively. Leadership must set the tone for an inclusive and equitable workplace by modelling the behaviours they wish to see. This includes fostering an environment where all employees, regardless of their background, feel respected, valued, and supported in their professional journeys. By committing to these changes, the pharmacy profession can begin to dismantle the systemic barriers that continue to hold back women of colour, particularly Black women, and create a more inclusive future for all.

Anti-blackness and colourism

Anti-Black racism is a critical factor behind the alarming disparities faced by Black people in Great Britain, where they are disproportionately subjected to police stop-and-search practices compared to their white and Asian counterparts. This over-policing is only one aspect of the systemic challenges that Black communities confront. In addition, Black individuals are disproportionately affected by issues such as homelessness, poverty, and unemployment. These inequalities are not random; they are deeply rooted in historical prejudices that trace back to the brutal legacy of slavery and colonialism. During these periods, Black people were systematically dehumanised and portrayed as inferior and lazy—a narrative that continues to inform racist attitudes today. However, it is important to acknowledge that anti-Black racism is not exclusive to white individuals. Harmful beliefs about Black people are also perpetuated by people of other ethnic backgrounds, such as in South Asian communities[41], demonstrating that anti-Blackness is a pervasive issue across multiple communities.

The use of broad terms like BAME or POC (People of Colour) has become common in discussions about race and discrimination. While these terms may offer a convenient shorthand for referring to non-white groups, hence the use of the terms in this book, they often mask the unique and disproportionately negative experiences that Black people face. The lived realities of Black individuals, as supported by data, are distinct from those of other ethnic minorities and are often far more severe. Grouping all minority ethnic experiences together under one umbrella risks erasing the specific forms of racism that target Black people. It is crucial, therefore, to recognise the distinctiveness of anti-Black racism and to address it in a way that acknowledges these specific experiences rather than generalising them under a single, broad category of racial discrimination.

Even within the Black community, experiences of racism are not uniform. There are varying degrees of discrimination based on skin tone, a phenomenon known as colourism. Black individuals with lighter skin often experience different forms of bias compared to their darker-skinned counterparts. Those with lighter skin may find it easier to gain acceptance in certain societal and professional spaces, while those with darker skin often face harsher discrimination. This colourism extends into the professional world, including in fields such as pharmacy, where white and Asian individuals disproportionately fill leadership roles. This trend suggests that colourism and skin colour bias may play a role in the underrepresentation of Black individuals in leadership positions within the profession.

If a comprehensive survey were conducted in the pharmacy profession, it would likely reveal significant gaps created by colourism and skin colour bias. These gaps are likely to be evident in areas such as pay disparities, recruitment, retention, and overall experiences of racial discrimination. Even existing data, such as the Pharmacy Workforce Race Equality Standard (WRES) report, provides a glimpse into these inequities. The report groups various ethnicities under the BAME label, but even within this broad categorisation, the data shows that there was a marked underrepresentation of BAME staff in higher-paid roles in 2022. However, the report fails to explore how this underrepresentation specifically affects individuals with darker skin tones or those who identify as Black. By not disaggregating the data, the report misses a critical opportunity to uncover the full extent of racial disparities within the profession, particularly the impact of colourism. Have you ever been the only Black person employed in an almost entirely Asian department, as I was during my time at the RNOH? If so, was your experience positive or as challenging and isolating as mine? These are the kinds of experiences that need to be explored, documented and reported to truly understand how colourism contributes to perpetuating racial discrimination within the pharmacy profession. The reality is that working or studying in an ethnically diverse environment does not guarantee a safe space when it comes to racial discrimination.

Addressing these issues requires more than just acknowledging that disparities exist. It demands targeted actions aimed at dismantling the systemic barriers that disproportionately disadvantage Black individuals. This includes confronting the intersection of racism and colourism, particularly in professions like pharmacy, where, in my view, these biases impact recruitment, retention, and progression. Institutions must commit to data transparency, ensuring that reports like WRES do not obscure the nuanced and often more severe experiences of Black individuals by grouping all ethnic minorities together. Moreover, organisations must develop and implement policies that specifically address anti-Black racism and colourism, ensuring that Black professionals, particularly those with darker skin, are not only represented but also equitably compensated and supported throughout their careers.

It has been argued that society operates within an invisible "Hierarchy of Race and Acceptance Pyramid" (figure 9). This pyramid illustrates how perceived skin colour correlates with levels of social acceptance. This concept arranges racial and ethnic groups with lighter-skinned individuals at the top, descending to those with darker skin tones. The pyramid helps explain why people with lighter skin are often more readily accepted by society than those with darker complexions.

Belief in this concept can shed light on how colourism and systemic racial bias influence perceptions of credibility, belonging, and opportunity. It is a powerful reminder of the implicit and explicit hierarchies that remain embedded within social, professional, and institutional environments, highlighting the ongoing need for intersectional strategies to promote equity and inclusion.

Do you recognise this hierarchy in your workplace or educational setting? If not, perhaps you are fortunate to be in a truly inclusive environment. An environment where leadership reflects the diversity of the pharmacy profession and where there are opportunities to flourish. But if you do see this pyramid, ask yourself why it exists. More importantly, consider what actions you are prepared to take to address it. After all, inaction is a choice, and it, too, carries consequences.

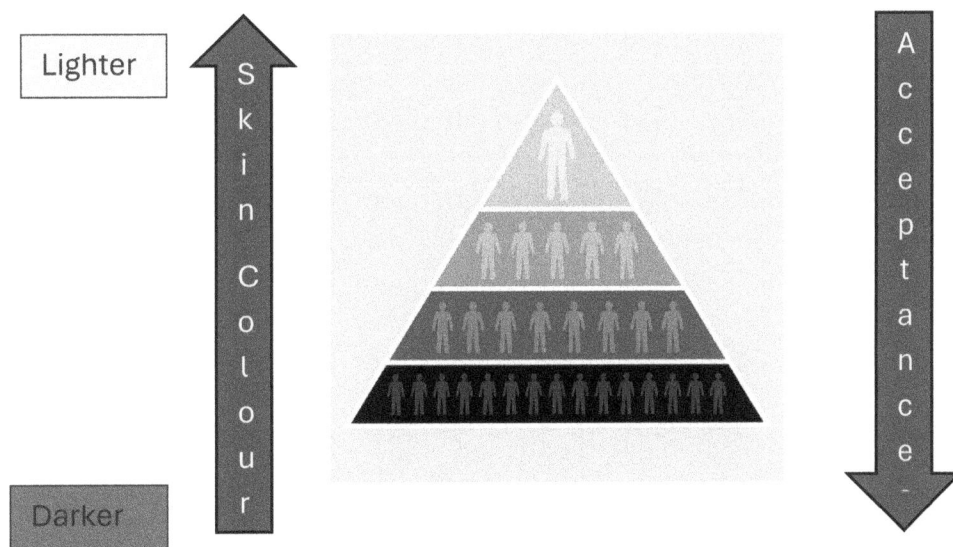

Figure 9: Skin Colour vs Social Acceptance Hierarchy.

Overall, the fight against anti-Black racism and colourism is a crucial step toward achieving true equity in society and in professional sectors like pharmacy. It is essential to recognise the specific challenges that Black individuals face, both within and outside the workplace, and to implement targeted strategies that address these challenges head-on. Only by doing so can we begin to dismantle the systemic barriers that continue to marginalise and disadvantage Black people in Britain today.

References

41. Sivathasan, N., South Asian anti-black racism: 'We don't marry black people', A. Network, Editor. 2020: BBC NEWS.

Chapter Six: Leadership, Tokenism and Representation in Pharmacy

The pharmacy "Colour of Power"

"The Colour of Power" is a comprehensive research project by "Operation Black Vote," in partnership with the Guardian newspaper and Green Park recruitment, examining who holds top positions across key public, private, and democratic institutions in the UK[42] The findings reveal a stark reality: pathways to the highest roles remain largely inaccessible for Britain's BAME communities.

In 2017, the study found that only 3.4% of the 1,049 top jobs were occupied by BME individuals, meaning 97% of Britain's most powerful roles were held by white individuals. The research spanned 37 sectors, highlighting the persistent lack of diversity in positions of influence across the nation.

Despite public commitments from government, public bodies, and businesses to enhance diversity at leadership levels, progress has stagnated. According to the latest research from Green Park, this slow change continues to characterise the UK's leadership landscape. "The Colour of Power 2020" update visualises the diversity—or lack thereof—among Britain's key decision-makers, showing that just 52 of the top 1,099 roles (or 4.7%) are held by non-white individuals. This modest increase of only 1.2% (or 15 additional roles for ethnic minorities) since the 2017 index is a sobering reminder of the enduring challenges to representation and equity despite a non-white population representing 13% of the UK.

The data underscores the need for more effective, sustained efforts to break down systemic barriers and build inclusive pathways to leadership.

In the context of the pharmacy profession, which stands as the third largest healthcare profession in the UK, there are striking parallels with the findings of "The Colour of Power" project. Between October and November 2024, I looked up the photos of those appointed or selected to executive and leadership roles in the following pharmacy organisations:

- **Department of Health and Social Care**: Responsible for setting national health and social care policy and overseeing the NHS in England.
- **NHS England, NHS Scotland and NHS Wales**: Responsible for delivering and overseeing health services in their respective nations, each operating independently with devolved powers to set healthcare policy, budgets, and service priorities.
- **General Pharmaceutical Council**: Regulator for pharmacists, pharmacy technicians and pharmacies in Great Britain.
- **Royal Pharmaceutical Society**: Leads the profession of pharmacy in Great Britain.

- **Association of Pharmacy Technicians UK**: The professional leadership body for UK pharmacy technicians.
- **Pharmacy Defence Association**: Support the needs of pharmacists in the UK. When necessary, it defends their reputation.
- **Guild of Healthcare Pharmacists**: Defends the interests of pharmacists working in hospitals, primary care and other healthcare institutions for the NHS and commercial healthcare providers in the UK.
- **The National Pharmacy Association**: Supports independent community pharmacies in the UK to succeed professionally and commercially for the benefit of their patients.
- **Boots Pharmacists Association**: Trade Union that supports Boots pharmacists.
- **British Pharmaceutical Students' Association**: The official student organisation of the Royal Pharmaceutical Society.
- **Academy of Pharmaceutical Sciences**: The professional body for scientists in the UK involved in research and development activities associated with medicines, medical devices and diagnostics.
- **Community Pharmacy England**: The representative body for all community pharmacy owners in England.
- **Pharmacist Support**: An independent charity supporting pharmacists and their families, former pharmacists, trainee pharmacists and pharmacy students.
- **Association of the British Pharmaceutical Industry (ABPI)**: Represent companies which invest in making and discovering medicines and vaccines.

After careful reflection, I made the decision not to publish the images I gathered for this book out of respect and for ethical and legal boundaries surrounding image rights and consent. Nevertheless, assembling those visuals was a profoundly emotional experience, which was marked by sadness, frustration, and a deep sense of urgency. The impact of these images is difficult to articulate; it is only by seeing them side by side that one fully grasps the stark reality they depict. I therefore encourage the reader to undertake a simple yet revealing exercise: create a visual collage of what I call the "Pharmacy Colour of Power." Include as many key figures as possible, such as Chief Pharmacists, Superintendent Pharmacists, and senior pharmacy leaders from both public and private sectors. In doing so, you will begin to see a pattern. The racial and ethnic composition of pharmacy leadership speaks volumes about the persistent disparities in representation. The predominance of lighter skin tones among decision-makers exposes a clear and troubling lack of ethnic diversity at the highest levels of influence within the profession. This silent visual narrative is a powerful reminder that equity in pharmacy is still a work in progress and one we must actively and collectively pursue.

Furthermore, when confronted with the overwhelming lack of visible diversity among senior pharmacy leaders, one cannot help but question whether being a person of colour, particularly being Black, presents a barrier to ascending into decision-making roles within the profession. This observation is not made to discredit the accomplishments or qualifications of those currently in leadership; I have no doubt that many have earned their positions through dedication, skill, and merit. Yet, the recurring overrepresentation of Caucasian professionals at the highest levels of pharmacy leadership prompts a deeper examination of the structural and systemic factors that shape access to these roles. Why are so few racially minoritised professionals represented in spaces where policies are made, budgets are allocated, and strategic visions are formed? Why do we rarely see Black pharmacists in executive, superintendent, or chief pharmacist positions across sectors? These patterns suggest not just an individual shortfall but a broader institutional failure to nurture, promote, and include diverse talent. It calls for honest dialogue, accountability, and a commitment to dismantling the invisible barriers that continue to limit representation and perpetuate inequality in our profession.

Among all the organisations I examined, the British Pharmaceutical Students' Association (BPSA) stood out as the only one that truly reflected the ethnic diversity of both the pharmacy profession and the UK. The BPSA Board embodies a range of ethnic backgrounds, showcasing the talent and potential within the field. Unfortunately, for many of these students, who have demonstrated remarkable leadership skills from the very beginning of what should be a promising career, their role at the BPSA may be the only leadership position they ever hold in pharmacy.

It's a stark and disheartening reality: despite their drive and contributions, many talented individuals face barriers that prevent them from advancing within the profession. This underrepresentation isn't just an individual loss; it's a missed opportunity for the profession to benefit from diverse perspectives, experiences, and innovations that could shape the future of pharmacy. The lack of pathways for these skilled young professionals raises serious concerns about inclusivity and equity within our field, leaving a generation of potential leaders sidelined.

Importance of diversity in decision-making positions

Race and ethnic diversity in decision-making positions are vital for fostering equity, innovation, and cultural competence within any organisation or field, particularly in healthcare and pharmacy.

The patterns of racial discrimination observed in healthcare, from unethical medical experiments like the Tuskegee Study to the forced sterilisation of minority women, also manifest in the pharmaceutical world. Just as racial biases have influenced medical research and patient care, they have shaped how medications are developed, tested, and distributed, perpetuating inequalities in treatment outcomes for minority populations. These biases extend into the pharmacy profession, where racial disparities in drug prescribing, patient interactions, and workforce equity persist.

Racial inequality within the pharmacy industry is reflected not only in patient care but also in the experiences of minority pharmacists themselves. The 2023 Pharmacy WRES report revealed that Black pharmacy staff were three times more likely to report experiencing workplace discrimination compared to their White colleagues. This discrimination affects career progression, job satisfaction, and workplace morale, reinforcing systemic barriers for ethnical minority professionals in the field.

Additionally, wage disparities further illustrate these inequalities. A salary survey conducted by the *Pharmaceutical Journal* between April 15 and April 30, 2024, revealed a median pay gap of 7.2% between white pharmacists and those from ethnic minority backgrounds, with white pharmacists earning a median hourly wage of £29.20 compared to £27.10 for minority pharmacists. This gap, which was 7.3% in 2021, shows little sign of closing, highlighting persistent economic inequality in the profession[43].

These disparities in both treatment and opportunity underscore how racism pervades all sectors of healthcare, including pharmacy. Addressing these inequalities requires systemic changes at multiple levels, including policy reform, better representation of minority groups in decision-making positions, and targeted efforts to close wage gaps and eliminate workplace discrimination. Without such efforts, the profession risks perpetuating the same historical inequities seen across the broader healthcare.

Having diverse perspectives in leadership positions can mitigate the risks of implicit and explicit biases affecting decisions. By bringing in leaders who can speak to different lived experiences, organisations can challenge stereotypes and avoid one-size-fits-all approaches to policies or patient care.

Especially in fields like healthcare, where patient relationships are paramount, a diverse leadership team demonstrates a commitment to social responsibility and aligns the organisation with the values of the community it serves.

Tokenism

In 2020, after the racially motivated killing of George Floyd in the United States, there was an unprecedented outpouring of activism against racism worldwide. Organisations around the world made sure they communicated their stance against racism. Many of these organisations did not have Black representation in their leadership, so they went on to employ Black people into leadership positions. It really felt as if racism was going to be taken seriously and change was going to start happening at last.

Moving forward to 2025, little change has happened. If anything, we seem to be going back to what things used to look like before the death of George Floyd. Organisations did not change. It seems that it was a mere tokenism exercise to hire a handful of Black people into leadership positions with no intention of changing services, processes or outcomes.

The truth is that tokenism is not an appropriate or effective approach to addressing racial inequality because it focuses on superficial actions rather than genuine, meaningful change. Tokenism involves making quick or symbolic efforts to appear inclusive, often by recruiting a small number of people from underrepresented groups to give the illusion of diversity without addressing the underlying systemic issues.

The problem with tokenism is that it fails to address systemic inequality. It does not address the root causes of racial inequality within an organisation. Simply hiring a few individuals from minority groups without challenging or changing the policies, practices, and culture that perpetuate inequality does nothing to dismantle systemic racism. True racial equality requires a deep commitment to overhauling organisational structures, such as fair hiring, promotion processes, and equitable access to resources and opportunities. Token hires may lead to short-term appearances of diversity, but they don't result in long-term, structural change.

Tokenism can create an environment where individuals from underrepresented groups who are hired may feel isolated, undervalued, or even exploited. This creates a hostile and unwelcoming environment for those individuals who are brought into a workplace that has not genuinely embraced inclusivity. Without a doubt, those individuals will find themselves sidelined, unsupported, and expected to represent or "prove" their entire demographic group. This can create feelings of alienation and additional stress for these individuals, as they are often left to navigate an environment that is not truly inclusive or supportive of their success.

Furthermore, rather than challenging and breaking down harmful stereotypes, tokenism can inadvertently reinforce them. When people from underrepresented groups are hired as symbolic gestures, it implies that their presence is for show rather than due to their qualifications, skills, or potential. This can lead to the perception that they are only in their roles because of their race or background rather than being valued contributors to the organisation. As a result, tokenism can reinforce biased assumptions and stereotypes rather than dispel them.

We need to ask ourselves if tokenism hinders progress toward diversity and inclusion in the pharmacy profession by allowing organisations to claim they are addressing the issue without making substantive efforts. This gives the illusion of progress while concealing ongoing problems, such as a lack of representation in leadership, pay disparities or unequal opportunities for advancement. When organisations use token hires to signal a commitment to diversity, it detracts from the need for genuine, long-term initiatives that aim to create an equitable and inclusive environment for all employees. Apart from not resulting in any meaningful progress, I suspect that tokenism is leading to disillusionment and frustration among both minority and majority pharmacy professionals. Minorities may feel they are being used to satisfy diversity quotas or to improve the public image of the organisations rather than being appreciated for their contributions. Majorities may also perceive token hires as unfair or dismiss the importance of diversity, seeing these efforts as purely symbolic. In both cases, the result is an erosion of trust and morale within the workplace. Overall, tokenism reduces the impact of genuine diversity by merely meeting numeric goals without creating an environment where diverse voices are heard, respected and valued. By focusing on appearances, tokenism prevents organisations from fully realising the benefits that come with true inclusivity and a diverse workforce.

Black and Brown faces in high places

Despite the clear disadvantages of tokenism, the fact is that it will continue to take place, resulting in a minority of Black and Brown women and men sometimes employed in leadership positions. However, those who rise through the ranks and, with their actions or inactions, perpetuate the same racial harm that has historically been inflicted pose a serious danger to efforts toward equality. By doing so, they provide institutions with a convenient "get-out-of-jail-free card", allowing these organisations to point to their diversity without addressing the deeper issues of systemic racism and inequality. By trying to fit within the organisation's culture, you often see these Black and Brown individuals being reluctant to challenge policies and practices that are not inclusive or are discriminatory. As a consequence, these individuals often become complicit in upholding structures of oppression, validating the status quo while neglecting the real work of dismantling discriminatory practices. Their presence can mask institutional failures, giving the false impression of progress while racial harm persists unchallenged. In the pharmacy context, where Black leaders are scarce, particularly at the national level, this can be damaging and dangerous.

Unlike medics and nurses, pharmacy professionals in the UK have rarely engaged in meaningful activism to address racial inequalities. There's often a reluctance rooted in the belief that pharmacy is somehow immune to these issues or that its professionals are not the recipients of racial discrimination. I understand that perspective. Still, despite my own experiences, I don't define myself as a victim. On the contrary, I see myself as someone who has endured injustice and chosen to confront and overcome it with the courage to speak out, even when it comes at a cost.

I remember clearly when the Pharmacy WRES was released. Its arrival was met with silence and no widespread debate, just carefully worded PR statements from a few national organisations. Aside from a blog I wrote for *Chemist and Druggist*, there was little public commentary. It felt as though no one really cared. But change doesn't happen in silence. Activism requires activists, people moved by their own experiences of inequality, discrimination, or marginalisation, who are willing to speak up and act. Without that drive, progress remains performative, not transformative.

Life experiences often lead to a deeper awareness of societal issues. I know this from my personal experience of racism in the pharmacy profession. I believe that those who have encountered systemic barriers firsthand, like I have, are likely to become more educated about the root causes of inequality and the need for structural reform. This knowledge fuels activism as people seek to address the gaps in policies, systems, and cultural practices perpetuating injustice. So the question is why, in the pharmacy profession, where there is racial discrimination, we don't see activism by those who have experienced it? I don't believe that those who have moved up to higher positions have not experienced racial discrimination. So why don't they use their position to amplify the voices of marginalised peers who are often silenced or ignored? After all, leaders have the power to enact structural and policy changes within organisations and governments.

BAME pharmacy leaders can push for organisational policies that promote equality, diversity, and inclusion. This includes advocating for fair hiring practices, pay equity, and unbiased promotion processes that ensure equal opportunities for all employees, regardless of their racial or ethnic background. BAME pharmacy leaders can also work to establish policies that protect employees from discrimination and microaggressions, creating a more inclusive workplace culture.

One of the most powerful ways BAME pharmacy leaders can improve racial inequality is by amplifying the voices of those who are marginalised. They can use their platforms to bring attention to the challenges faced by minority groups and create space for these individuals to share their experiences. By doing so, they ensure that the needs and concerns of BAME employees and communities are heard and addressed.

Role of authentic activism in combating racism in pharmacy

Activism is essential in combating racial inequality, as it raises awareness, challenges systemic injustices, and drives social and institutional change. It mobilises people to take collective action, demanding equal rights, fair treatment, and accountability from governments, organisations, and institutions. As a catalyst for policy reform, activism puts pressure on leaders to implement legislative changes that dismantle discriminatory practices and promote racial equity. Historical movements like "*Black Lives Matter*" and the civil rights struggles of the past have demonstrated the power of activism in changing laws, reshaping public discourse, and broadening the understanding of justice.

In the workplace, activism pushes organisations to adopt inclusive practices, implement diversity and equality initiatives, and hold leadership accountable for creating truly representative and supportive environments. It is vital to dismantle institutional racism by challenging biased hiring practices, pay disparities, and decision-making processes that disproportionately affect people of colour.

It is often said that it should not be the responsibility of people of colour to fix racism, as they are not the ones who caused it. However, non-white leaders play a critical role in addressing and improving racial inequality within organisations and society at large. Their lived experiences, cultural insights, and leadership positions uniquely position them to advocate for meaningful change and create inclusive environments. These leaders serve as role models, showing that individuals from underrepresented backgrounds can succeed in leadership roles, thereby challenging stereotypes and inspiring others from minority communities to aspire to similar positions. Moreover, they can mentor and support emerging talent, building a pipeline of future leaders from diverse backgrounds. Abandoning this responsibility is not only irresponsible but a missed opportunity to drive real progress.

That said, activism must be intentional and authentic. It should not be used to elevate the social profile of individuals seeking power without substance or results. Empty activism achieves little and yields no meaningful impact. In pharmacy, we need leaders who can demonstrate tangible actions that have positively transformed the experiences of those facing discrimination. Activism should not solely focus on reducing workplace discrimination but also on improving health outcomes for marginalised communities.

For example, how many pharmacy professionals have identified the over-prescribing of antipsychotics in Black men or the under-prescribing of pain relief for Black patients, raised these issues with prescribers, and advocated for changes in practice? This includes implementing guidelines that ensure ethnicity is considered when prescribing. I know that even when I was aware of these issues, I never fully addressed the relationship between ethnicity and prescribing practices. I may have intervened to adjust doses, but I never felt confident in raising broader systemic concerns. However, our profession should be doing more to address health inequalities and improve outcomes. Pharmacists, whether in the community or hospital settings, are well-placed to tackle these disparities, but as a profession, we often shy away from such opportunities.

I believe we would feel more empowered to confront these challenges if our professional, commissioning, and regulatory bodies took a stronger, more active stance on addressing these critical issues. The need for pharmacy professionals to lead meaningful change, both in reducing discrimination and in advancing equitable health outcomes, is long overdue. However, without leadership that genuinely reflects the increasingly diverse population of the UK, such change may feel like a distant ideal rather than an achievable reality.

References

42. Tulsiani, R. The Colour of Power. 2020 [cited 2024; Available from: https://www.green-park.co.uk/insight-reports/the-colour-of-power/s191468/..

43. Burns, C. and D. Connelly. *What will it take to fix pharmacy's stubbornly unchanged ethnicity pay gap?* [cited 2025 January, 19]; Available from: https://pharmaceutical-journal.com/article/feature/what-will-it-take-to-fix-pharmacys-stubbornly-unchanged-ethnicity-pay-gap.

Chapter Seven: Patient Care and Racial Bias in Pharmacy

Impact of racism on patient treatment and medication access

Racism, whether conscious or unconscious, can lead to biased clinical decisions, resulting in unequal treatment for patients from marginalised racial or ethnic groups. Healthcare professionals may, even unintentionally, hold assumptions about pain tolerance, disease susceptibility, or treatment adherence based on race. This unequal treatment can lead to suboptimal care and poorer health outcomes for affected patients.

As discussed earlier, racial minorities are often underrepresented in clinical trials, which can limit the understanding of how different populations respond to medications. This lack of representation affects the development of treatments that are effective and safe across diverse populations, leading to one-size-fits-all approaches that may not address the unique needs of certain racial or ethnic groups.

In pharmacy settings, bias may affect how pharmacy professionals interact with patients, including their willingness to provide detailed counselling or go the extra mile to ensure access to high-cost medications. Moreover, systemic racism can influence broader healthcare policies and funding allocations, leading to under-resourced healthcare facilities in predominantly minority communities and limiting their access to both healthcare professionals and medications.

Worldwide, structural racism, including socioeconomic inequalities and discriminatory policies, often limits access to necessary medications. Minority populations may experience financial barriers, a lack of health insurance, or restricted access to pharmacies and healthcare facilities. Even when medications are available, cost can become a prohibitive factor, disproportionately affecting lower-income patients who are more likely to belong to marginalised racial groups. This can delay treatment and worsen disease progression.

Over time, the compounded effects of racism in treatment decisions, medication access, and overall care contribute to stark disparities in health outcomes for minority populations. Conditions like hypertension, diabetes, and cancer often see higher rates of morbidity and mortality among racial minorities, in part due to delays in receiving proper treatment or medication.

Addressing the impacts of racism on patient treatment and medication access requires a multi-faceted approach, including educating healthcare professionals on implicit bias, improving access to healthcare in underserved communities, and ensuring diversity in clinical trials and health policy development.

Case studies of unequal care

Pharmacy services are placed at the heart of the community. They are easily accessible to the wider population. In secondary and tertiary care, pharmacy professionals work collaboratively with the multidisciplinary team. This puts pharmacy professionals in an ideal position to intervene and prevent unequal care due to ethnicity across various healthcare systems.

There are several case studies and research findings that highlight unequal care due to ethnicity. These disparities exist in access to care, quality of treatment, patient outcomes, and even the diagnosis and management of medical conditions.

Maternal care

In both the United States and the United Kingdom, Black women are significantly more likely to die from pregnancy-related complications than white women. In the U.S., Black women are three to four times more likely to die from childbirth or pregnancy-related causes[44]. In the UK, Black women are five times more likely to die during childbirth. Contributing factors include systemic racism, bias in healthcare settings, lack of access to prenatal care, and a general lack of responsiveness to the concerns of Black women in medical settings. Research has shown that healthcare professionals may dismiss or minimise Black women's pain and symptoms, leading to delayed treatment or mismanagement of complications[2]. Serena Williams, the world-renowned tennis player, nearly died from post-birth complications[45]. Despite the clear communication of her symptoms, her concerns were initially dismissed by medical professionals, highlighting the broader issue of how even high-profile women can experience unequal care.

Covid - 19

During the COVID-19 pandemic, people from BAME communities in the UK and racial minorities in the U.S. experienced disproportionately higher rates of infection, hospitalisation, and death compared to white populations. These disparities were linked to several factors, including higher exposure risks due to socioeconomic conditions (e.g., frontline jobs), underlying health conditions, limited access to healthcare, and delayed or inadequate care. There was also evidence of unequal treatment, with some reports of BAME patients being denied critical care interventions or receiving care later than white patients. Public Health England's review showed that Black and Asian people were more likely to die from COVID-19, prompting calls for urgent changes in healthcare access and treatment to address these systemic issues[46].

During the pandemic, countless frontline staff lost their lives, with a disproportionate number coming from BAME backgrounds. Among those who tragically succumbed to the virus while providing essential services were pharmacy professionals such as Pooja

63

Sharma, Jayesh Patel, Mehool Patel, Jermaine Wright, and Mandy Siddorn. Their dedication to serving their communities cost them their lives.

As President of the UK Black Pharmacists Association (UKBPA), I was deeply shocked and saddened by the messages I received from Black pharmacists during this uncertain period. At a time when compassion was desperately needed, I witnessed an alarming rise in racism within the profession. One particular case that stood out was that of a pregnant Black pharmacist working in a Clinical Commissioning Group (CCG). She messaged me to tell me she was threatened by her white female line manager with redeployment to the NHS Nightingale Hospital in London unless she agreed to move to a community pharmacy role. NHS Nightingale London was the first of several temporary hospitals set up by NHS England specifically to treat COVID-19 patients. This Black pharmacist was being forced to choose between two patient-facing roles, one working in a community pharmacy and the other facing the risk of exposure to COVID-19 at a hospital treating COVID-19-positive patients. Meanwhile, her white colleagues were all assigned to remote work from home.

Another example involved a Black foundation year student working in the Intensive Care Unit (ICU) when COVID-19 hit. Despite having completed his ICU rotation, he was asked to repeat it, while a white student who was due to rotate into the ICU was instead allowed to stay in a non-COVID ward.

In January 2020, I was working one day a week at an NHS Trust in Essex. On one occasion, an Asian pharmacist failed to visit a ward with a suspected COVID-19 patient on the day she was scheduled. She told the pharmacy technicians that I could visit the ward the next day when I was due to be on duty. Upon arrival, the pharmacy staff informed me of the situation. Initially, I thought there might have been a misunderstanding, but it became clear that I was being asked to visit her ward after completing my own. I politely refused and submitted my notice when both the Asian Deputy Chief Pharmacist and the white Chief Pharmacist disregarded my concerns. I concluded that what was not safe for them was not safe for me.

In response to these troubling events, I began investigating what could be done to address the systemic issues at play. I attended meetings with several pharmacy organisations. On June 12, 2020, the Royal Pharmaceutical Society (RPS) and the UKBPA launched a survey aimed at assessing the safety of pharmacists and pre-registration students during the pandemic[47]. The survey sought to determine whether employers had implemented risk assessments and made necessary adjustments to the working environment to safeguard pharmacy teams. The results were staggering: 78% of Black pharmacists and pre-registration students felt they were at an increased risk of contracting COVID-19 and believed that changes to their working conditions were essential[48]. This survey was launched nearly two months after NHS England had issued a letter on April 29, 2020, advising NHS organisations to carry out risk assessments for staff at higher risk of contracting COVID-19[49].

These findings highlighted the deeply rooted inequalities within the pharmacy profession and the urgent need for change to ensure the safety and well-being of all pharmacy professionals, particularly those from BAME backgrounds.

Pain Management

Numerous studies have shown that Black patients are systematically undertreated for pain compared to white patients. One significant study in 2016 found that medical students and residents in the U.S. were more likely to underestimate the pain of Black patients and were less likely to recommend adequate pain relief[50]. The underlying false beliefs, such as Black patients having "thicker skin" or a higher pain tolerance, contribute to this unequal care. In one particular study, Black children were significantly less likely to receive pain medication for appendicitis in emergency rooms compared to white children, highlighting a consistent trend of racial bias in pain management[51].

Mental Health

Ethnic minorities are often underserved in mental health care, receiving less treatment or lower-quality care than their white counterparts. In the UK, Black men are more likely to be diagnosed with schizophrenia and are disproportionately sectioned under the Mental Health Act while being less likely to receive community-based mental health care[52, 53]. In the U.S., African-American and Hispanic populations are less likely to receive mental health treatment and are more likely to be misdiagnosed[54]. Contributing factors include stigma, cultural misunderstandings, lack of access to culturally competent care, and provider bias. A study in the UK showed that Caribbean and Black African patients with mental health conditions are more likely to be detained involuntarily and less likely to be referred to community-based therapy or psychological interventions. This has led to higher rates of involuntary hospitalisation and severe treatment outcomes[55].

Diabetes Management

African American and Hispanic patients in the U.S. are less likely to receive timely or adequate diabetes care compared to their white counterparts. This includes delays in diagnosis, lower rates of receiving standard care (such as HbA1c monitoring, foot exams, and eye checks), and worse health outcomes, such as higher rates of complications, including amputations and kidney disease. Disparities in diabetes care are often tied to socioeconomic factors, insurance status, language barriers, and implicit bias from healthcare providers. Studies have shown that African American patients with diabetes are more likely to have worse glycaemic control than white patients, even when accessing similar healthcare settings, suggesting that provider bias and treatment disparities play a significant role[56, 57].

In the UK, the *"Tackling Inequality Commission Report"* showed that individuals of Black and South Asian ethnicity are less likely to receive access to the latest treatments compared to their white counterparts. Similarly, people from ethnic minority backgrounds or those living in deprived areas are less likely to use life-changing technologies like wearable glucose monitors or insulin pumps for managing diabetes. Despite their transformative potential, these advancements remain inaccessible to many due to systemic inequalities. Ethnic minorities and those facing socioeconomic challenges face significant barriers, limiting their ability to benefit from innovations that could greatly improve their health and quality of life[58].

Cancer Care

Ethnic minorities often receive later-stage cancer diagnoses and less aggressive treatment compared to white patients. For example, Black men in the U.S. are more likely to be diagnosed with prostate cancer at an advanced stage and are less likely to receive optimal treatment[59]. In the UK, similar patterns are seen with breast cancer and cervical cancer screenings, where women from ethnic minorities are less likely to receive early detection and timely treatment[60]. These disparities are driven by barriers to healthcare access, socioeconomic factors, cultural mistrust of the healthcare system, and racial bias in healthcare settings. A U.S. study found that African American women with breast cancer were less likely to be offered breast-conserving surgery and were more likely to receive suboptimal care. Similarly, Hispanic women were less likely to receive timely chemotherapy for breast cancer compared to white women[61-64].

Sickle Cell

Sickle Cell Disease (SCD), which primarily affects people of African and Caribbean descent, is often underfunded and under-researched compared to other genetic disorders like cystic fibrosis, which predominantly affects white populations. In both the U.S. and the UK, SCD patients report being undertreated for pain crises and facing scepticism from healthcare providers regarding the severity of their symptoms[65, 66]. The disparity in care and research investment is often attributed to racial bias and the systemic neglect of diseases primarily affecting minority populations. In the UK, patients with sickle cell disease reported facing longer waits for treatment in emergency departments compared to patients with other conditions, reflecting systemic bias and inadequate care[67].

The death of Evan Nathan, a 21-year-old British Black man who died on the 25th of April 2019 at North Middlesex Hospital in Edmonton because of staff ignoring the symptoms of a sickle cell crisis, is an example of how tragic health outcomes can be for ethnic groups[68].

Again, on the evening of 30th December 2023, Dave Onawelo, 34, died in a London hospital waiting room after staff failed to recognise the severity of his condition. A coroner's report revealed that Dave, who had sickle cell disease, sought help at Whipps Cross Hospital after struggling to breathe. Despite telling staff he believed he was experiencing a sickle cell crisis, partial observations deemed him not acutely unwell, and he was left waiting. His condition deteriorated, and staff initially dismissed his mother's concerns. When finally attended to, Dave was critically anaemic, acidotic, and had dangerously low blood sugar. Attempts to resuscitate him failed, and he died of acute respiratory failure, acute chest syndrome, and complications from sickle cell disease[69].

The coroner criticised the hospital for failing to identify and treat a critically ill patient, noting issues like hospital overcrowding and the staff's lack of clinical curiosity and compassion. Proper care could have saved Dave's life.

HIV

In the United Kingdom, African immigrants represent a significant proportion of people living with HIV. Many African immigrants face unique challenges that lead to poorer health outcomes compared to native-born white patients with HIV. African immigrants are often diagnosed at later stages of HIV infection. In London in 2016, late diagnoses were reported in 61% of Black African men and 52% of Black African women, compared to 48% of white heterosexual men, 42% of white heterosexual women, and 24% of gay or bisexual men[70]. These may be that many African immigrants face barriers to accessing healthcare, such as lack of knowledge about available services, fear of deportation, and stigma associated with HIV. These barriers result in lower rates of engagement with HIV care services. Also, stigma within African communities, combined with racism in healthcare systems, contributes to delays in seeking care and difficulty in adhering to treatment regimens. African immigrants are less likely to achieve viral suppression, which is critical for improving health outcomes and reducing the transmission of HIV. All of the above results in African immigrants living with HIV in the UK having higher rates of morbidity and mortality compared to their white counterparts.

The role of pharmacy professionals in addressing racial disparities in patient outcomes

Pharmacy professionals play a crucial role in addressing racial disparities in patient outcomes, as the ones described above, by promoting equitable healthcare access, optimising medication management, and advocating for culturally competent care. Their direct interactions with patients and involvement in care decisions uniquely position them to bridge healthcare gaps for minority populations.

One significant way pharmacy professionals can improve patient outcomes is by delivering culturally competent services. Recognising the diverse needs and challenges faced by different racial and ethnic groups includes understanding cultural beliefs about health and medication, respecting language preferences, and being aware of how different communities perceive the healthcare system. By enhancing communication and building trust, pharmacy professionals can help minority patients better understand their treatments and adhere to medication regimens. This can involve offering multilingual medication instructions or utilising translation services to ensure patients with limited English proficiency have a clear understanding of their care.

Minority populations often experience lower medication adherence due to factors like limited access, high costs, mistrust in the healthcare system, and insufficient patient education. Pharmacy professionals are already addressing these barriers by providing personalised patient counselling, collaborating with prescribers to identify affordable alternatives (such as generic medications), and educating patients on the importance of medication adherence. They also help navigate prescription assistance programs and suggest cost-effective options, tackling the financial obstacles that disproportionately affect racial and ethnic minorities.

But they can do more. Additionally, pharmacy professionals can advocate for expanded healthcare access in underserved communities. This can include supporting telepharmacy and mobile pharmacy services to reach patients who face geographical or socioeconomic barriers. By pushing for policy changes and investing in community outreach, pharmacists can help improve healthcare infrastructure in areas where it is most needed.

It is essential to stop viewing pharmacy professionals merely as a resource to alleviate the burden on busy doctor clinics. With adequate funding and government support, pharmacy professionals can play a more active role in community education and health promotion, especially in minority communities with historically limited access to healthcare information. By hosting health workshops, distributing educational materials, and offering preventive services like screenings and immunisations, they can enhance health literacy and encourage early intervention for conditions that disproportionately impact racial minorities, such as hypertension, diabetes, and sickle cell disease. For example, conducting educational campaigns about blood pressure monitoring in Black communities can help prevent severe complications associated with uncontrolled hypertension.

Furthermore, pharmacy professionals can contribute to reducing racial disparities by collecting and analysing data on patient outcomes, medication use, and health inequities. This data-driven approach allows for the identification of trends and gaps in care, enabling the implementation of targeted interventions. For instance, pharmacy professionals can analyse local prescription patterns to detect racial or ethnic disparities in treatment—such as lower rates of cholesterol-lowering medications prescribed to Black patients—and take steps to address these inequities.

The COVID-19 pandemic underscored the lower vaccination uptake rates in minority populations, driven by mistrust, access challenges, and misinformation. Pharmacy professionals played a vital role in addressing these disparities by promoting and administering vaccines in underserved communities. By setting up local clinics, combating vaccine hesitancy, and providing accurate information about vaccine safety, the profession helped improve vaccination rates and public health outcomes for BAME communities.

Overall, pharmacy professionals can make a meaningful impact in addressing racial disparities in healthcare through culturally competent care, policy advocacy, reducing access barriers, and engaging in patient education and chronic disease management. Their close proximity to patients and expertise in medication therapy management empower them to promote health equity and reduce disparities effectively.

The importance of cultural sensitivity in patient care

Cultural sensitivity is essential in patient care because it directly impacts the quality of care delivered, builds patient trust, and leads to improved health outcomes. By acknowledging and respecting patients' diverse cultural backgrounds, beliefs, and practices, healthcare providers can offer more personalised and effective treatment.

Firstly, cultural sensitivity significantly enhances communication and understanding. Miscommunication is more likely to occur when healthcare providers and patients do not share the same language or cultural norms, resulting in potential misunderstandings about diagnoses, treatment plans, or medication instructions. When providers invest effort into understanding a patient's cultural context, it fosters trust and openness. This, in turn, encourages patients to share vital information, adhere to treatment plans, and feel comfortable asking questions.

Furthermore, patients are more likely to trust and feel at ease with healthcare providers who respect their cultural background. Trust is a cornerstone of effective healthcare, influencing patients' willingness to disclose sensitive information and follow medical guidance. On the other hand, culturally insensitive interactions can lead to feelings of alienation or fear, causing patients to delay seeking care or withhold important health details.

Cultural sensitivity also plays a vital role in reducing health disparities, which are often exacerbated by cultural misunderstandings, socioeconomic factors, and systemic biases. By offering culturally sensitive care, healthcare providers can address these barriers and deliver more equitable treatment, especially for minority and marginalised populations. This approach helps reduce the disproportionate disease burden experienced by these groups.

Additionally, culturally sensitive care can lead to better health outcomes. When treatment plans incorporate cultural beliefs and practices—such as dietary restrictions, religious practices, customs, or traditional healing methods—patients are more likely to adhere to their prescribed regimens. This alignment with cultural values promotes adherence to treatment and preventive measures, ultimately enhancing overall health. For instance, Diabetes UK provides culturally tailored dietary recommendations, including dishes like "Jollof rice", vegetable "Chow Mein", and "Channa Dahl", to support healthier eating habits for diabetic patients from diverse backgrounds[71].

Another significant benefit of cultural sensitivity is its ability to reduce bias and stereotyping. Recognising each patient as an individual with unique cultural experiences allows healthcare providers to avoid assumptions and deliver unbiased, respectful care. This approach minimises the risk of misdiagnoses or inappropriate treatment, which can be especially detrimental to minority populations.

Respecting patients' values and beliefs is a fundamental component of cultural sensitivity. Many patients have culturally influenced views on health and healing, such as the preference for family involvement in medical decisions or adherence to spiritual practices. By honouring these beliefs, healthcare providers show that they value the patient's perspective, fostering a more collaborative and effective treatment process. When patients feel welcome and respected in an inclusive environment, they are more likely to have positive healthcare experiences and feel a greater sense of belonging within the healthcare system. This inclusivity benefits individual patients and contributes to improved public health outcomes.

As healthcare becomes increasingly globalised, cultural sensitivity enables providers to adapt to the needs of diverse populations. Pharmacy is often the first port of call for those seeking medical treatment. Therefore, it is paramount that pharmacy professionals understand cultural nuances to deliver appropriate and effective care. This adaptability is crucial for those serving immigrant and refugee communities, where cultural understanding can make a significant difference in patient outcomes. By incorporating cultural factors into the decision-making process, healthcare providers can engage in a collaborative approach that respects patient values, leading to higher patient investment in their care and greater satisfaction with treatment.

Cultural sensitivity is also critical in addressing mental health stigma within diverse communities. Mental health issues are often heavily stigmatised in many cultures, making it difficult for individuals to seek help. A culturally sensitive approach can help normalise mental health treatment, encouraging patients to access support in ways that align with their cultural beliefs. Tailored mental health interventions can break down these barriers, making care more accessible and respectful.

Educating healthcare professionals on cultural sensitivity is crucial, and there are many resources available to support this education. The Centre for Pharmacy Postgraduate

Education (CPPE) provides valuable resources on cultural sensitivity, emphasising the importance of continuous learning and practice in this area[72].

References

44. Harper, M., et al., *Why African-American women are at greater risk for pregnancy-related death.* Annals of Epidemiology, 2007. **17**(3): p. 180-185.

45. Gardner, S. *Serena Williams describes a near-death experience she had after giving birth to daughter Olympia.* [cited 2025 January, 18]; Available from: https://eu.usatoday.com/story/sports/tennis/2022/04/07/serena-williams-near-death-childbirth-complications/9504616002/.

46. Mackey, K., et al., *Racial and ethnic disparities in COVID-19–related infections, hospitalizations, and deaths: a systematic review.* Annals of Internal Medicine, 2021. **174**(3): p. 362-373.

47. Risk assessment survey for pharmacists launched. Available at: https://www.pharmacy.biz/coronavirus/risk-assessment-survey-for-pharmacists-launched/.

48. Coronavirus: 70% of BAME pharmacists have had no risk assessment - survey. Available at: Coronavirus: 70% of BAME pharmacists have had no risk assessment - survey - BBC News.

49. Second phase of the NHS response to COVID-19. Available at: https://www.england.nhs.uk/coronavirus/wp-content/uploads/sites/52/2020/04/second-phase-of-nhs-response-to-covid-19-letter-to-chief-execs-29-april-2020.pdf.

50. Hoffman, K.M., et al., *Racial bias in pain assessment and treatment recommendations, and false beliefs about biological differences between blacks and whites.* Proceedings of the National Academy of Sciences, 2016. **113**(16): p. 4296-4301.

51. Goyal, M.K., et al., *Racial disparities in pain management of children with appendicitis in emergency departments.* JAMA pediatrics, 2015. **169**(11): p. 996-1002.

52. Halvorsrud, K., et al., *Ethnic inequalities and pathways to care in psychosis in England: a systematic review and meta-analysis.* BMC Medicine, 2018. **16**: p. 1-17.

53. Bignall, T., et al., *Racial disparities in mental health.* Race Equality Foundation, 2019.

54. Blumberg, S.J., T.C. Clarke, and D.L. Blackwell, *Racial and ethnic disparities in men's use of mental health treatments.* 2015.

55. Solanki, J., L. Wood, and S. McPherson, *Experiences of adults from a Black ethnic background detained as inpatients under the Mental Health Act (1983).* Psychiatric Rehabilitation Journal, 2023. **46**(1): p. 14.

56. Oldroyd, J., et al., *Diabetes and ethnic minorities.* Postgraduate medical journal, 2005. **81**(958): p. 486-490.

57. Rodríguez, J.E. and K.M. Campbell, *Racial and ethnic disparities in prevalence and care of patients with type 2 diabetes.* Clinical Diabetes, 2017. **35**(1): p. 66-70.

58. DiabetesUK. *Tackling Inequality Commission Report.* 2023; Available at: https://www.diabetes.org.uk/sites/default/files/2023-11/366_Tackling_Inequality_Commission_Report_DIGITAL%20(1).pdf.

59. Chornokur, G., et al., *Disparities at presentation, diagnosis, treatment, and survival in African American men, affected by prostate cancer.* The Prostate, 2011. **71**(9): p. 985-997.

60. Bolarinwa, O.A. and N. Holt, *Barriers to breast and cervical cancer screening uptake among Black, Asian, and Minority Ethnic women in the United Kingdom: evidence from a mixed-methods systematic review.* BMC Health Services Research, 2023. **23**(1): p. 390.

61. Thompson, B., et al., *Breast cancer disparities among women in underserved communities in the USA.* Current breast cancer reports, 2018. **10**: p. 131-141.

62. Fazeli, S., et al., *Access to Breast Cancer Screening: Disparities and Determinants—AJR Expert Panel Narrative Review.* American Journal of Roentgenology, 2024.

63. Li, C.I., K.E. Malone, and J.R. Daling, *Differences in breast cancer stage, treatment, and survival by race and ethnicity.* Archives of internal medicine, 2003. **163**(1): p. 49-56.

64. Miranda, P.Y., W. Tarraf, and H.M. González, *Breast cancer screening and ethnicity in the United States: implications for health disparities research.* Breast cancer research and treatment, 2011. **128**: p. 535-542.

65. Haywood Jr, C. et al., *The impact of race and disease on sickle cell patient wait times in the emergency department.* The American Journal of Emergency Medicine, 2013. **31**(4): p. 651-656.

66. Pulte, D., et al., *Comparison of emergency department wait times in adults with sickle cell disease versus other painful etiologies.* Hemoglobin, 2016. **40**(5): p. 330-334.

67. Kmietowicz, Z., *Patients with sickle cell disease are let down by lack of coordinated NHS care, report finds.* 2023, British Medical Journal Publishing Group.

68. Mahase, E., *Sickle cell disease: inquiry finds serious care failings and racism towards patients.* 2021, British Medical Journal Publishing Group.

69. Willis, A. *Man, 34, dies in London hospital waiting room 2 hours after staff ignore accurate self-diagnosis.* 2024 [cited 2025 January, 19]; Available from: https://www.mylondon.news/news/health/man-34-dies-london-hospital-29895883.

70. Fakoya, I., et al., *HIV testing and sexual health among black African men and women in London, United Kingdom.* JAMA network open, 2019. **2**(3): p. e190864-e190864.

71. DiabetesUK. *Ethnicity and type 2 diabetes*. [cited 2025 January, 19]; Available from: https://www.diabetes.org.uk/about-diabetes/type-2-diabetes/diabetes-ethnicity.

72. CPPE. *Cultural competence hub*. [cited 2025 January, 18]; Available from: https://www.cppe.ac.uk/services/cultural-competence.

Chapter Eight: Solutions and Strategies for Anti-Racism in Pharmacy

Initiatives for creating a more inclusive and equitable pharmacy profession

In July 2018, the PDA BAME Network launched the ground-breaking PDA Anti-Racist Pharmacy Toolkit[73]. This toolkit was designed to assist PDA members, PDA representatives, and other pharmacists in identifying and addressing potential issues of racism within their workplaces. It provides practical steps and resources for determining whether racism exists in a given environment and offers signposts to help individuals resolve these issues. Importantly, the toolkit focuses on promoting racial equality for all members, ensuring that race-related concerns are addressed in a proactive and structured manner.

The toolkit was developed in collaboration with pharmacy professionals, academics, and policy advisors alongside the PDA, the only independent trade union exclusively for pharmacists in the UK. Its creation was not just an academic exercise—it was a deliberate, necessary response to the real and ongoing challenges faced by BAME individuals within the pharmacy profession. The toolkit also serves as a critical resource for trade union activists, providing them with the tools they need to engage in open and productive conversations about racial inequality in the workplace. It offers a foundation for activists to build local campaigns, advocate for change, and negotiate meaningful improvements in their work environments.

The PDA Anti-Racist Pharmacy Toolkit emphasises that identifying racism requires vigilance, especially in its more subtle forms. For example, if pharmacists are being treated unfairly or discriminated against—whether overtly or indirectly—due to their race, then racism is clearly present. Furthermore, if an employer is not actively taking steps to create an equitable and inclusive work environment, such as by addressing biases in recruitment practices, promoting BAME representation in leadership, or providing adequate EDI training, then these omissions suggest that racism still persists. The toolkit encourages the review and modification of workplace structures to ensure that all workers, regardless of race, can operate in a fair and supportive environment.

The toolkit begins by providing clear definitions of key terms, helping users understand the various ways racism can manifest in the workplace. From there, it offers a step-by-step guide to addressing racism, from recognising discriminatory practices to building coalitions for change. Its ultimate goal is to empower pharmacists and their representatives to create workplaces where all employees feel valued and included, free from the toxic effects of racial bias.

Although the frequency of the toolkit's use and its overall impact have not been formally reported to my knowledge, the mere existence of this comprehensive resource is reassuring. Knowing that pharmacy professionals have access to a structured, supportive framework to navigate and challenge racism is a crucial step toward building a more equitable profession. The PDA Anti-Racist Pharmacy Toolkit serves as both a practical tool and a symbol of the ongoing commitment of the PDA to eradicate racism within the pharmacy, providing a much-needed platform for sustained dialogue and action on this critical issue.

Moving forward, assessing the toolkit's reach and effectiveness will be important. Gathering feedback from PDA members who have used it could offer valuable insights into its impact on workplace culture and whether further adaptations or additions are needed. The long-term goal is not just to respond to instances of racism but to foster a culture within the pharmacy profession that actively promotes equality and inclusion, ensuring that no one is left behind due to their race or ethnicity.

Regulatory changes needed to combat racism in pharmacy

A report by the General Medical Council (GMC) titled "*Equality, Diversity and Inclusion Targets, Progress and Priorities for 2024*" highlights the significant challenges faced by British doctors of BAME origin and overseas-trained medics working in the UK[74]. In the report, the GMC warned of the "persistent and pernicious" inequality these doctors endure throughout their careers. According to the findings, doctors from BAME backgrounds are disproportionately reported for alleged misconduct compared to their white British-trained peers. Many also encounter "discrimination and disadvantage" as they attempt to advance in their medical careers, with some areas of the NHS described as having a hostile "culture."

Bravo to the GMC for highlighting that inequality affects doctors at every stage of their journey, from education and training to senior leadership roles. These longstanding, deeply rooted issues negatively impact morale and hinder doctors' performance, prompting the GMC to advocate for equal and fair treatment for all medical professionals, regardless of background. As they emphasise, this systemic unfairness not only harms individuals but also tarnishes the reputation of health services. "Fair treatment is a right for all doctors, not just a select few," the GMC states.

Meanwhile, the GPhC has developed an EDI strategy aimed at combating various forms of discrimination within the pharmacy profession. The goal is to foster an inclusive culture where pharmacy teams feel empowered to fulfil their professional and legal obligations[75]. In 2022, the GPhC convened a roundtable with key stakeholders from the pharmacy sector to discuss how racism affects pharmacists and pharmacy technicians, along with the subsequent impact on patient care[76]. Despite these initiatives, critics argue that the GPhC's actions may be more performative than substantive.

For years, the GPhC has failed to meet Standard 15 of the Professional Standards Authority for Health and Social Care (PSA), which pertains to the timeliness of fitness-to-practise (FTP) investigations[77]. This shortcoming disproportionately impacts BAME pharmacy professionals, who are subjected to investigations more frequently than their white counterparts. The GPhC itself has acknowledged that Asian and Black pharmacists are overrepresented in FTP concerns. In 2021/2022, all non-white ethnic groups, except those identifying as mixed race or preferring not to disclose their ethnicity, were overrepresented in FTP cases.

The data reveals that Asian pharmacists comprised 38% of the GPhC register but accounted for 46% of FTP concerns and 52% of investigations. Black pharmacists made up 7% of the register yet were the subject of 10% of FTP concerns and investigations. In contrast, white pharmacists represented 42% of the register but were involved in only 24% of FTP concerns and 21% of investigations[78]. These statistics suggest a troubling disparity, with BAME pharmacists facing a greater likelihood of being referred to and undergoing FTP procedures.

In November 2024, it was reported that the GPhC carried out a grossly incompetent investigation. As a result, a High Court judge ordered the GPhC to re-open an investigation into a pharmacist over fraud allegations after "grossly incompetent errors" by the regulator caused him to believe for almost a year that the case had been dropped [79].

Lengthy and delayed investigations exacerbate the negative impact on BAME professionals' well-being, not to mention the financial burden of legal defence, particularly if the referral is racially motivated and unrelated to professional competency. For the GPhC to genuinely combat racial discrimination, it must address these delays and hold individuals accountable for racially motivated referrals. Proven instances of racially driven actions should result in immediate suspension and removal from the register. The GPhC must advocate a zero-tolerance policy toward racism—anything less amounts to mere performative gestures.

Best practices for addressing and preventing racism in the pharmacy profession

Dismantling systemic racism in pharmacy requires a comprehensive approach that includes diversifying the workforce, reforming education and hiring practices, addressing patient care disparities, advocating for policy change, and fostering a culture of accountability. By taking these steps, the pharmacy profession can help build a more inclusive, equitable, and effective healthcare system for all patients, regardless of their race or ethnicity.

An essential first step in creating a fair and inclusive recruitment process is raising awareness and addressing biases in hiring practices. This can be achieved by improving the recruitment process to make it genuinely blind, using diverse interview panels, and establishing clear, objective criteria for evaluating candidates and their performance. Having specific and unambiguous assessment criteria is crucial; otherwise, the absence of such standards allows for biased recruitment practices to flourish and become ingrained. It is important to recognise that looking at candidates' GPhC registration numbers during shortlisting to infer their identities does not constitute a blind process. Additionally, having non-ethnically diverse panels interviewing a group of ethnically diverse candidates can disadvantage those who are not represented on the panel. To mitigate this, panels should be composed of members from various departments and include members of the public. This approach helps to reduce biases and promote a fair evaluation process. Concerns such as "the job was already given before the interview" highlight the perception that hiring decisions are sometimes made during the shortlisting phase, with interviews conducted solely to fulfil legal requirements. Addressing these practices by ensuring transparency and fairness in recruitment is critical to building a more equitable hiring environment.

Creating a comprehensive, ongoing strategy that fosters an inclusive and equitable environment is the only acceptable approach to addressing and preventing racism in pharmacy. Leadership plays a pivotal role in this effort. Pharmacy leaders must be visibly committed to championing anti-racism initiatives, not just during symbolic moments like *"Black History Month"* but all year round. Too often, the responsibility of organising diversity-related events is relegated to Black staff during these designated times, which reinforces the problem rather than addressing it. Leaders should consistently communicate the importance of EDI and lead by example. They must be held accountable through measurable goals and regular reporting on EDI initiatives, with key performance indicators (KPIs) related to diversity and inclusion integrated into their evaluations. A critical question is: What are leaders doing to increase the representation of marginalised groups, particularly in leadership roles? Research shows that diverse leadership can better reflect and address the needs and concerns of underrepresented employees and patients. There must also be a clear, zero-tolerance policy for racism, with consistent consequences for those who engage in racist behaviour, enforced uniformly across the organisation.

Education is another key pillar in combating racism within the pharmacy profession. Awareness of how racism manifests in healthcare should start in pharmacy schools and continue throughout professional life. This goes beyond merely decolonising the curriculum; it requires implementing compulsory, ongoing training in unconscious bias, cultural competence, and anti-racism for all pharmacy professionals. Additionally, training should focus on the mental and physical effects of microaggressions, helping individuals recognise these subtle but harmful behaviours. Understanding their signs and symptoms is crucial for creating a more inclusive and supportive work and studying environments.

Pharmacy professionals must also be empowered to act when they witness racism or discrimination. Active bystander training should be integral to professional development, equipping staff with the skills and confidence to intervene when they encounter racism. Furthermore, anonymous and safe reporting channels must be available for professionals to report incidents without fear of retaliation. A clear, unbiased process for investigating these complaints is essential, as self-investigation often leads to complaints being dismissed and racist practices becoming institutionalised. Failing to address these issues properly sends the message that reporting discrimination is futile. Following a complaint, there must be a follow-up process to ensure that the affected individuals receive adequate support and that the issue is fully resolved. Continuous employee feedback should be used to refine and improve the complaint process, ensuring transparency and accountability.

Data-driven approaches are vital for addressing and preventing racism in pharmacy. Tracking and analysing diversity metrics must be integrated into institutional strategies. Continuous data collection on hiring, promotions, pay equity, and retention rates by race and ethnicity provides tangible insights into race relations within the profession. This data helps identify disparities and allows for the monitoring of EDI initiatives' effectiveness, enabling organisations to make necessary interventions. Regular assessments of institutional culture and employee experiences related to diversity and inclusion are crucial for maintaining an accurate pulse on the workplace climate. Pharmacy institutions must be willing to adapt their strategies based on what is or isn't working, using real-time data to guide adjustments.

Addressing and preventing racism in pharmacy requires long-term commitment and sustained efforts. EDI initiatives should not be viewed as one-off projects but as ongoing, evolving processes. For the sustainability of the profession, we must view equality, diversity and inclusion as essential components of a thriving healthcare system. Only by embedding these principles into the core of our profession can we ensure a truly equitable future for all pharmacy professionals.

Pulse Surveys, which are short, frequent surveys, allow organisations to regularly assess the experiences of their employees, providing real-time insights into workplace culture and identifying issues related to discrimination. They are powerful tools for monitoring racial discrimination in the workplace. By providing regular, anonymous feedback, these surveys help organisations identify trends, measure the success of EDI initiatives, and hold leadership accountable for creating an inclusive environment. When used effectively, pulse surveys allow organisations to address racial discrimination in real time, fostering a culture of openness, transparency, and continuous improvement.

The role of pharmacy leaders and educators in shaping a more inclusive future

Pharmacy leaders and educators have a unique and influential role in shaping a more inclusive future by promoting diversity, addressing health inequities, developing inclusive policies, and educating the next generation of pharmacy professionals to be more culturally competent and equity-focused. Through these efforts, they can help build a pharmacy profession that is not only clinically excellent but also socially responsible and responsive to the needs of all patients.

A crucial role is ensuring that the profession is representative of the diverse communities it serves. By promoting diversity in recruitment, education, and leadership, they can help create a workforce that understands the unique challenges faced by different populations, leading to more culturally sensitive and patient-centred care. Leaders should not just advocate but also prove that they observe inclusive hiring practices, mentorship programs, and leadership pathways for underrepresented groups.

By integrating inclusivity into the curriculum, educators can ensure students are not only well-versed in clinical and technical knowledge but also understand health disparities, social determinants of health, and cultural competence. This prepares future pharmacists to recognise and address the unique needs of marginalised communities, such as ethnic minorities, the LGBTQ+ population, and individuals with disabilities. Incorporating case studies that reflect diverse patient populations and teaching students to recognise and mitigate biases in treatment will foster more empathetic and equitable care practices in the pharmacy profession.

Pharmacists are expected to examine medications and their use. As part of the multidisciplinary healthcare teams, they are placed in a unique position to influence policies and practices that reduce health inequities. They can work with healthcare organisations, policymakers, and other stakeholders to develop strategies that improve access to medications and healthcare services for underserved populations. This includes addressing barriers like cost, language, and geographic location, as well as advocating for changes in healthcare policy that prioritise equity. Pharmacy leaders can also spearhead initiatives that focus on preventative care, chronic disease management, and education in communities that face health disparities.

An example of how pharmacy can address language barriers is *Written Medicine*[80], a mission-driven solution enterprise. It was created to address the communication and language barriers that exist between healthcare providers and patients. The online medical translation solution and terminology service improve medication adherence, clinical safety, patient independence and safety. Founded by pharmacy manager Ghalib Khan in 2012, Written Medicine aims to improve medication adherence and reduce health inequalities by removing communication barriers between pharmacists and patients.

Finally, both pharmacy leaders and educators can serve as mentors and role models, demonstrating the values of inclusivity, empathy, and respect for diversity. By mentoring the next generation of pharmacy professionals, leaders can instil a commitment to equity and inclusion from the earliest stages of their careers. Encouraging young pharmacy professionals to pursue leadership roles in advocacy and community health can help sustain long-term change in the profession.

True allyship in combating racial discrimination in pharmacy

Allyship in racial discrimination involves actively supporting and advocating for marginalised racial groups by recognising and addressing racial inequalities. True allyship goes beyond passive support, requiring continuous learning, reflection, and action.

An ally listens to the experiences of marginalised individuals, acknowledging their perspectives and pain without judgment or defensiveness. They create a space for open dialogue and genuinely try to understand the impact of racism. Allies take responsibility for educating themselves about racial issues and histories rather than relying on people of colour to explain racism. They read, watch, and listen to resources that offer insight into systemic racism and oppression. Allies leverage their own privilege to highlight the voices and concerns of those affected by racial discrimination, whether by speaking out in meetings, sharing content from minority voices, or advocating for change within institutions. An ally actively confronts and calls out racist behaviour or language, whether it's overt or subtle. They don't wait for others to take action and address microaggressions, biases, or discriminatory policies directly. Allies engage in advocacy consistently, not just during high-profile incidents of racial injustice. They support policies and initiatives that address structural racism and work to create inclusive environments, even when it may be uncomfortable or inconvenient. Allies are self-aware and introspective, acknowledging their own biases and working to unlearn them. They view this as an ongoing journey, understanding that they may make mistakes but are committed to improving.

Posting a statement or image on social media without any sustained commitment to anti-racist action is performative. Allyship is not about appearing virtuous but about making tangible contributions to fighting discrimination. Allyship is not about "rescuing" marginalised people or speaking over them. True allies recognise that people facing racial discrimination are the best advocates for their own experiences and work collaboratively rather than assuming a leadership role over the affected group. A genuine ally does not become defensive when confronted with their own biases or privileged perspectives. Allies understand that learning involves being open to criticism and viewing it as a chance to grow, not something to dismiss. Allies do not seek attention or applause for their actions. Instead, they focus on supporting others and elevating the voices of those historically marginalised, letting them lead the conversation. Allyship is not a one-time action; it's a continuous process. Attending one protest, reading one book, or making one donation without ongoing engagement and learning does not constitute true allyship. Allyship isn't just interpersonal; it includes advocating for structural change within institutions, policies, and laws. Simply being "kind" to individuals is not enough if an ally isn't also working to dismantle the systemic structures that perpetuate racial inequality. True allies never dismiss or downplay the experiences of racism shared by others. They do not say things like, "I don't see colour," or "Racism doesn't exist here," as these statements invalidate others' lived realities.

In Summary, real allyship requires intentional action, continuous education, and humility. It's about advocating for those affected by racial discrimination both in private and public, supporting systemic change, and understanding that true progress takes time and consistent effort.

References

73. PDABAME *PDA Anti-Racist Pharmacy Toolkit*. 2022. Available from: https://www.the-pda.org/wp-content/uploads/Anti-racist-Toolkit-FINAL.pdf'.

74. .GMC, *Equality, diversity and inclusion Targets, progress and priorities for 2024*. 2024: Available at: https://www.gmc-uk.org/-/media/documents/equality-diversity-and-inclusion---targets-progress-and-priorities-for-2024_pdf-108776261.pdf.

75. .GPhC. *Delivering equality, improving diversity and fostering inclusion. Our strategy for change 2021–26*. 2021 [cited 2025 January, 19]; Available at: https://assets.pharmacyregulation.org/files/document/gphc-equality-diversity-inclusion-strategy-november-2021.pdf.

76. GPhC. *Racism in pharmacy: report on the roundtable event* 2022 [cited 2025 January, 19]; Available at: https://assets.pharmacyregulation.org/files/document/racism-in-pharmacy-short-report-roundtable_event-november-2022-.pdf.

77. PSA. *General Pharmaceutical Council (GPhC) Performance Review – The monitoring year 2023/24* September 2024; Available at: https://www.professionalstandards.org.uk/sites/default/files/attachments/Monitoring%20report%20GPhC%202023-24.pdf.

78. Clews, G. *Asian and black pharmacists overrepresented in fitness-to-practise concerns, GPhC finds*. 2023 [cited 2025 January, 18]; Available at: https://pharmaceutical-journal.com/article/news/asian-and-black-pharmacists-overrepresented-in-fitness-to-practise-concerns-gphc-finds.

79. .Walsh, A., *Judge orders 'incompetent' GPhC to reopen export fraud allegations*. 2024, Communications International Group: Pharmacy Magazine.

80. Khan, G. *Written Medicine.* 2012 [cited 2025 19/01/2025]; Available at: https://writtenmedicine.com/.

Conclusion

Summary of key points

In the pharmacy profession, disparities exist in several key areas, including access to education and training, bias within the curriculum, and the subtle yet harmful discrimination and bullying faced by the workforce. These issues create unequal opportunities for individuals from underrepresented groups, limiting their advancement and fostering a culture where biases persist. Addressing these disparities requires targeted efforts to ensure equal access to education, eliminate curriculum biases, and create an inclusive, respectful work environment where all individuals are treated fairly and supported in their professional development.

Addressing racial discrimination in pharmacy requires an intersectional approach that considers how race intersects with other identities, such as gender, religion, disability, and sexual orientation, to address the inequities present in the profession fully. By recognising these intersections, pharmacy organisations can implement more comprehensive diversity and inclusion strategies considering the full scope of individuals' identities and experiences.

Addressing the issue of colourism is also important within the broader discussion of racial equity in pharmacy. Colourism—where individuals with lighter skin are often afforded more privilege—perpetuates inequality within communities of colour. Pharmacy institutions must ensure that anti-colourism policies are included in their EDI efforts, recognising that the experiences of Black women with darker skin may differ significantly from those with lighter skin tones. Addressing this issue head-on is crucial for creating an equitable and inclusive profession.

Pharmacy professionals who hold multiple marginalised identities (e.g., race, gender, disability) face compounded forms of discrimination, making it harder for them to advance, receive recognition, or feel included in the workplace. The underrepresentation of POC, particularly in leadership roles, limits the visibility of intersectional challenges and perpetuates a cycle where their unique experiences are overlooked. Addressing racial discrimination in pharmacy requires an intersectional approach that considers how race intersects with other identities, such as gender, disability, and sexual orientation, to fully address the inequities present in the profession.

Integrity and a non-political environment are essential for fostering a positive, collaborative and productive workplace culture. This would build trust, enhance collaboration, improve morale, encourage innovation, attract and retain talent, boost productivity, strengthen leadership, ensure fairness, aid in compliance and risk management and contribute to sustainable organisational growth.

Prioritising these values is crucial for safeguarding patient safety and maintaining the integrity of the healthcare system. By addressing and eliminating collusion, we can create a more transparent, fair, and effective healthcare environment that truly prioritises patient care and employee well-being.

The pharmacy profession needs to do better to safeguard both the workforce and members of the public. Being inquisitive about the culture within different pharmacy workplaces and encouraging staff to denounce collusion without the fear of persecution will go a long way.

We must foster an environment where transparency and accountability are paramount. This includes implementing robust reporting mechanisms that protect whistleblowers, ensuring their concerns are heard and addressed without retaliation.

Additionally, we must prioritise continuous education and training on ethical practices and the importance of integrity in healthcare. Leaders should be trained to recognise and address signs of collusion and other unethical behaviours, promoting a culture of openness and trust.

Creating a supportive and inclusive workplace culture is also essential. Staff should feel valued and respected, knowing their wellbeing is a priority. This involves regular workplace culture assessments, supporting mental health and establishing clear policies against discrimination and harassment.

Moreover, there should be a commitment to regular audits, surveys and reviews of pharmacy practices to ensure compliance with ethical standards and professional guidelines. These audits and surveys should be transparent, and the findings should be used to make informed improvements.

By being proactive and dedicated to fostering a culture of integrity and support, we can create a safer, more ethical environment in the pharmacy profession. This not only safeguards the workforce but also ensures the highest standards of care for the public.

Speak Up: A call to action.

"One day, you will tell your story of how you overcame what you went through, and it will be someone else's survival guide". – Brene Brown

"Speak Up Pharmacy" available at **https://speakuppharmacy.org/**, is an innovative digital platform designed to address the underreporting and lack of research on the ways racial discrimination manifests within the pharmacy profession. The platform empowers users to anonymously report their experiences of discrimination, categorised by sector and geographical area, providing a safe and secure space to raise awareness about the challenges faced by marginalised groups.

Unfortunately, there is little to no accountability for racial discrimination in the NHS, where many pharmacy professionals are employed. Without realising it, individuals may find themselves working in environments rife with microaggressions and overt discriminatory behaviour. "Speak Up Pharmacy" aims to address this issue by offering a platform that generates comprehensive reports, highlighting patterns of discrimination across various organisations and regions. These reports provide users with valuable insights into which employers and institutions prioritise diversity, equity, and inclusion, enabling them to make more informed decisions about where to work or study. By crowdsourcing real-world experiences, "Speak Up Pharmacy" brings transparency to workplace environments, helping to mitigate the risks of encountering racial discrimination.

Beyond reporting, "Speak Up Pharmacy" encourages networking among users who have had similar experiences, recognising the isolation that often accompanies racial discrimination and its intersectionality with gender, disability, and other identities. This feature fosters a supportive community where individuals can connect, share resources, and collaborate on solutions, helping to combat the feelings of isolation and alienation that are often part of these experiences.

The platform not only raises awareness and provides transparency but also contributes to broader systemic change. By offering policymakers, researchers, and organisations valuable data, "Speak Up Pharmacy" enables targeted interventions to address workplace inequalities and promote diversity, equity, and inclusion.

Ultimately, "Speak Up Pharmacy" is more than just a reporting tool—it's a comprehensive resource for empowering individuals, building supportive networks, and driving positive change within the pharmacy profession, ensuring safer and more inclusive environments for professionals from all backgrounds.

Ten questions for group discussion

The topic of racial discrimination in pharmacy is crucial to address for fostering a fair and equitable profession. The ten questions below provide a foundation for open conversations about the experiences, challenges, and potential solutions related to racial inequity within the field. These questions encourage pharmacy professionals to reflect on issues such as education on health disparities, the impact of microaggressions, the role of leadership representation, and effective support for underrepresented groups. By engaging with these questions, participants can share personal insights, learn from others' experiences, and collectively explore ways to create a more inclusive and supportive environment for all. The aim is to spark meaningful dialogue that can lead to practical changes, empowering everyone within the pharmacy profession to reduce discrimination and promote diversity, equity, and inclusion.

1. How should pharmacy schools and training programs teach future pharmacists about racial discrimination and health disparities?
2. How do microaggressions impact the daily work experiences of people of colour in the pharmacy profession?
3. Can you share an example of a time you or someone else faced racial discrimination at work? How was it handled, if at all?
4. Do you feel that our pharmacy practice takes sufficient positive action to support underrepresented groups in achieving equal opportunities? If yes, please share examples. If not, please suggest areas where you believe further support is needed.
5. How does the lack of representation in leadership roles contribute to racial discrimination in pharmacy, and what can organisations do to promote diversity at higher levels?
6. How can allies, especially non-minority colleagues, practically help address racial discrimination in the workplace?
7. How can pharmacy organisations create meaningful EDI initiatives that effectively combat racism?
8. How can we ensure complaints of racial discrimination are taken seriously and dealt with appropriately by leadership?
9. How can women of colour in healthcare advocate for systemic changes without fear of retaliation or career damage?
10. What concrete steps have you taken to address racial discrimination within your institution?

Personal notes and reflection

Ten Practical Solutions for an Inclusive Pharmacy Practice

Creating a truly inclusive pharmacy practice requires intentional efforts and proactive strategies. The ten practical solutions below outline actionable steps that pharmacy teams can implement to foster a welcoming and supportive environment for both staff and patients. By prioritising diversity, equity, and inclusivity in every aspect of the workplace—from recruitment and onboarding to ongoing engagement and community outreach—pharmacies can cultivate a culture where everyone feels valued and empowered. Each of the ten solutions offers a practical approach to addressing inclusivity challenges, ensuring that pharmacy teams not only reflect the diverse communities they serve but also enhance patient care through a range of perspectives and experiences. Embracing these practices can help create a stronger, more cohesive team that's committed to equitable and accessible healthcare for all.

1. Onboarding Survey

Conduct a comprehensive onboarding survey for new hires to gauge their initial experience and ensure they feel welcomed, valued, and supported. This survey can provide insights into their first impressions and help identify areas for improvement in your onboarding process, particularly concerning inclusivity and accessibility.

2. Pulse Surveys

Regularly administer pulse surveys to gather ongoing feedback from all team members. These short, frequent surveys help monitor team sentiment, engagement, and inclusivity over time, allowing the pharmacy to quickly address any emerging issues and make necessary adjustments to foster a more inclusive workplace.

3. Diverse Recruitment Strategies

Implement recruitment strategies that reach diverse candidate pools, focusing on inclusive job descriptions, broadening outreach channels, and actively engaging with underrepresented communities. A diverse recruitment approach can help build a workforce that better represents the community served, bringing a range of perspectives to improve patient care. Include members of the community and members of the wider healthcare community. Ideally, the line manager should not be on the panel to avoid recruitment based on similarity or affinity bias.

4. Post-Interview Surveys

Introduce post-interview surveys for candidates to provide feedback on the interview process. This feedback can help assess whether candidates felt the process was fair, inclusive, and respectful. Insights gained can guide improvements in interview practices, making them more welcoming and equitable.

5. Bias Awareness Training

Offer regular training on recognising and mitigating bias for all staff members, including those involved in hiring and patient care. This training helps create awareness of unconscious biases that may affect decision-making, ensuring a more inclusive approach in both internal and patient-facing interactions.

6. Inclusive Language and Communication

Encourage the use of inclusive language and provide resources or guidelines on respectful communication practices. This ensures that all staff and patients feel acknowledged and respected, enhancing the inclusivity of the pharmacy environment.

7. Mentorship and Sponsorship Programs

Establish mentorship or sponsorship programs that support the professional development of underrepresented groups within the pharmacy team. Mentorship can provide guidance, foster growth, and build confidence, while sponsorship actively promotes team members' career advancement.

8. Flexible Work Policies

Create flexible work policies that accommodate different needs, such as varying schedules, religious observances, and family obligations. This flexibility helps support work-life balance and ensures that the workplace is accommodating for all team members.

9. Community Engagement Initiatives

Partner with local organisations to promote pharmacy careers within diverse communities and to better understand the needs of different patient groups. This engagement can inform the practice's approach to inclusivity and help ensure it is meeting the needs of the populations it serves.

10. Regular Inclusivity Audits

Conduct inclusivity audits to assess policies, practices, and the physical work environment. These audits can identify barriers to inclusivity, such as accessibility issues or unintended biases in policies, and inform necessary changes to foster an inclusive workplace culture.

Personal notes and reflection

Epilogue: Is racism really a problem in our profession?

Letter to *"The Pharmaceutical Journal"* - 23 October 2020[81]

I must comment on the perceptions of Elsy Gomez Campos, president of the UK Black Pharmacist Association, and Nigel Praities, who interviewed her for 'There are too many excuses justifying the unjustifiable', published in the August issue of The Pharmaceutical Journal.

Parities says the Black Lives Matter marches in the UK have led to "much soul-searching over the discrimination black people face in society". Most people I talk to are dismayed at the associated lawlessness, including attacks on police and damage to buildings and statues.

He also implies that black, Asian and minority ethnic (BAME) people are more susceptible to COVID-19 owing to inequality caused by societal discrimination. This is not the case; for example, some Asian groups are more prone to diabetes, and some African groups have sickle cell anaemia.

Practices also imply that the General Pharmaceutical Council (GPhC) is biased against BAME pharmacists in fitness-to-practise investigations. Surely, students fail the preregistration exam because they didn't meet the required standard, not because of the GPhC's bias.

Gomez Campos is concerned that BAME candidates are excluded from achieving office, but there have been many Asian presidents of the Royal Pharmaceutical Society (RPS). If BAME candidates apply and are not appointed, there must have been a stronger candidate.

Gomez Campos makes several sweeping statements such as "discrimination, isolation and inequality is happening daily"; "people [... are being] isolated, physically attacked and [having] their reputations destroyed"; and "serious problem in pharmacy." How can these comments be substantiated?

She also states that some black people are at a disadvantage because they have no family support networks here in the UK. Has she thought of overseas students who are here coping with the same issue?

The pharmacy culture she alludes to does not reflect my experience. I have never come across any discrimination. I have worked with black, white and Asian pharmacists in harmony. How can there be institutional racism when a substantial proportion of pharmacists seem to be Asian?

In the UK, I have appointed black candidates to senior positions. My workforce was mostly black when I worked in Africa. I did not discriminate against them; neither did they give me a hard time because I was English.

Gomez Campos says she does not want tokenism, but she seems to want preferential support for BAME students. She appears to pressure the RPS, the GPhC and pharmacy schools to tilt the slope of the playing field in their favour.

Looking for problems (particularly around race and gender) where they do not exist is common. Often, this can attract the law of unintended consequences.

David Norris, Fellow, Royal Pharmaceutical Society

Dear David,

Thank you for your letter. I am glad that in your personal experience, you have not witnessed any of your colleagues being subject to the discrimination described by Elsy in her interview, and it is good to hear about your fair approach as a manager. However, that does not mean that what Elsy describes does not exist or that her experience is not representative or valid for reporting in the journal.

Specifically, you question the mention of the impact of COVID-19 on BAME communities, but a recent review from Public Health England says that this may be explained by factors including "social and economic inequalities, racism, discrimination and stigma".

Of course, the overrepresentation of members of BAME pharmacists in fitness-to-practise proceedings and the ongoing differential in pass rates for the preregistration exam for black African candidates are complicated issues, but the latter was the subject of a report commissioned by the General Pharmaceutical Council in 2016, which said there were reports of "explicit prejudice and perceptions of implicit bias" against black students.

It is right that we continue to highlight both these issues in the journal, even if it sometimes makes for uncomfortable reading.

Best wishes,

Nigel Praities, executive editor, The Pharmaceutical Journal

I hope that David Norris and others who share his perspective will approach this book with an open mind and a willingness to consider experiences that may differ from their own. The question is not whether racism exists in the pharmacy profession but how we, as a collective, respond to the evidence of its presence.

Pharmacy, like every other sector in our society, does not operate in isolation. It is part of a broader system where inequities—racial and otherwise—still persist. While David's personal experiences may not include witnessing or experiencing discrimination, this does not invalidate the lived experiences of those who have. Recognising that disparity exists, even when it hasn't touched our own lives, is an essential step toward building a more inclusive profession.

Individuals who have not encountered systemic bias, career barriers, or stereotyping may not be fully aware of how identity shapes professional experiences. Their viewpoint is often shaped by the privileges afforded to them within a profession that has, historically, not consistently acknowledged or addressed such inequalities.

While many pharmacy professionals may recognise these issues privately, open conversations about racism and discrimination in the workplace can still be difficult. Silence, however, can unintentionally reinforce the very structures that uphold inequality. Addressing racism openly and constructively is critical—not to divide, but to create a shared understanding and accountability across the profession.

We must expect our professional bodies, including the General Pharmaceutical Council (GPhC), to take reports of discrimination seriously and treat them with the same weight as other forms of misconduct. Discrimination, like any breach of professional standards, has a direct impact on the safety, well-being, and professional development of pharmacists and students.

As Bell Hooks once said, *"All our silences in the face of racist assault are acts of complicity."* If we are to genuinely progress as a profession, we must be willing to engage in these difficult but necessary conversations. Acknowledging the problem is not an admission of personal failure—it is a commitment to collective improvement.

Ultimately, the aim is not to assign blame but to foster a pharmacy profession that supports and uplifts all its members, regardless of background. That starts with listening, learning, taking responsibility and demanding accountability as we work together across the profession toward meaningful change.

References

81. Norris, D., *Is racism really a problem in our profession?* The Pharmaceutical Journal, 2020. **305**(7942).

References

1. Francis, R., *Report of the Mid Staffordshire NHS Foundation Trust public inquiry: executive summary.* Vol. 947. 2013: The Stationery Office.

2. Kapadia, D., et al., *Ethnic inequalities in healthcare: a rapid evidence review.* 2022.

3. NHSE, *Pharmacy Workforce Race Equality Standard* 2023. Available at: https://www.england.nhs.uk/long-read/pharmacy-workforce-race-equality-standard-report/.

4. GPhC. The GPhC register as of 30 September 2023 - Diversity data tables. 2025 [cited 2025 20/01/2025]; Available at: https://view.officeapps.live.com/op/view.aspx?src=https%3A%2F%2Fassets.pharmacyregulation.org%2Ffiles%2F2024-01%2Fgphc-all-register-diversity-data-september-2023.docx&wdOrigin=BROWSELINK.

5. Poskett, J., *National types: The transatlantic publication and reception of Crania Americana (1839).* History of Science, 2015. **53**(3): p. 264-295.

6. Morton, S.G. and Combe, G., 1839. Crania Americana; or, a comparative view of the skulls of various aboriginal nations of North and South America: to which is prefixed an essay on the varieties of the human species. Philadelphia: J. Dobson; London: Simpkin, Marshall.

7. Villarosa, L., *Myths about physical racial differences were used to justify slavery—and are still believed by doctors today.* The New York Times, 2019.

8. Fiscella, K., et al., *Inequality in quality: addressing socioeconomic, racial, and ethnic disparities in health care.* Jama, 2000. **283**(19): p. 2579-2584.

9. Murthy, V.H., H.M. Krumholz, and C.P. Gross, *Participation in cancer clinical trials: race-, sex-, and age-based disparities.* Jama, 2004. **291**(22): p. 2720-2726.

10. Health, N.I.o.C. and H. Development, *Health disparities: Bridging the gap.* 2000: The Development.

11. Passmore, S.R., et al., *"My Blood, You Know, My Biology Being out There...": Consent and Participant Control of Biological Samples.* Journal of Empirical Research on Human Research Ethics, 2024. **19**(1-2): p. 3-15.

12. Obuobi, S., M.B. Vela, and B. Callender, *Comics as anti-racist education and advocacy.* The Lancet, 2021. **397**(10285): p. 1615-1617.

13. White, R.M., *Unraveling the Tuskegee study of untreated syphilis.* Archives of Internal Medicine, 2000. **160**(5): p. 585-598.

14. Baptiste, D.L., et al., *Henrietta Lacks and America's dark history of research involving African Americans.* Nursing open, 2022. **9**(5): p. 2236.

15. Cronin, M., *Anarcha, Betsey, Lucy, and the women whose names were not recorded: The legacy of J Marion Sims.* Anaesthesia and Intensive Care, 2020. **48**(3_suppl): p. 6-13.

16. Lawrence, M., *Reproductive rights and state institutions: The forced sterilization of minority women in the United States.* 2014.

17. Spector-Bagdady, K. and P.A. Lombardo, *US Public Health Service STD experiments in Guatemala (1946–1948) and their aftermath.* Ethics & Human Research, 2019. **41**(2): p. 29-34.

18. Moreno, J.D., 2013. *Undue risk: secret state experiments on humans.* Routledge.

19. Saint Jean, A., *Racial Disparities Within Black Maternal Health.* Antiblackness and the Stories of Authentic Allies: Lived Experiences in the Fight Against Institutionalized Racism, 2024: p. 283.

20. Garretson, D.J., *Psychological Misdiagnosis of African Americans.* Journal of Multicultural Counseling & Development, 1993. **21**(2).

21. Fu, Y., et al., *Interventions to tackle health inequalities in cardiovascular risks for socioeconomically disadvantaged populations: a rapid review.* British Medical Bulletin, 2023. **148**(1): p. 22-41.

22. Nazroo, J.Y., et al., *Ethnic inequalities in access to and outcomes of healthcare: analysis of the Health Survey for England.* Journal of Epidemiology & Community Health, 2009. **63**(12): p. 1022-1027.

23. Gadson, A., E. Akpovi, and P.K. Mehta. *Exploring the social determinants of racial/ethnic disparities in prenatal care utilization and maternal outcome.* in *Seminars in perinatology.* 2017. Elsevier.

24. Dreyer, B.P., *The toll of racism on African American mothers and their infants.* JAMA Network Open, 2021. **4**(12): p. e2138828-e2138828.

25. Mukwende, M. *Black & Brown Skin.* 2020 [cited 2025 20/01/2025]; Available at: https://www.blackandbrownskin.co.uk/.

26. Mukwende, M., *Mind the gap: A clinical handbook of signs and symptoms in black and brown skin.* Wounds UK, 2020. **16**(3): p. 16.

27. Shannon, L., *Subnormal: A British Scandal.* 2021, BBC: UK. Available at: https://www.bbc.co.uk/programmes/m000w81h.

28. Webster, D., *Is Uni Racist?*, in *Black & British.* 2021, BBC: UK. Available at: https://www.bbc.co.uk/programmes/p09dhr3f.

29. Doll, A., *Chasing Equality in Pharmacy Training–Closing the Awarding and Attainment Gap for Black Trainees in Pharmacy.* 2024.

30. Johnston, L., G. Cameron, and T. Vanson, *Qualitative research into Registration Assessment performance among Black-African candidates.* Report to the General Pharmaceutical Council.[Online] Accessed, 2016. **31**(01): p. 2018.

31. Greenwald, A.G. and M.R. Banaji, *Implicit social cognition: attitudes, self-esteem, and stereotypes.* Psychological Review, 1995. **102**(1): p. 4.

32. Cox, T. *The huge differences in racism in pharmacy between ethnicities.* 2020; Available at: https://www.chemistanddruggist.co.uk/CD005219/The-huge-differences-in-racism-in-pharmacy-between-ethnicities.

33. NHSE, *Medical Workforce Race Equality Standard (MWRES) 2020.* 2021. p. 29. Available at: https://www.england.nhs.uk/wp-content/uploads/2021/07/MWRES-DIGITAL-2020_FINAL.pdf.

34. NHSE, *NHS Workforce Race Equality Standard (WRES) 2022 data analysis report for NHS trusts*. 2023: NHSE. p. 43. Available at: https://www.england.nhs.uk/long-read/nhs-workforce-race-equality-standard-wres2022-data-analysis-report-for-nhs-trusts/.

35. Sue, D.W. and L. Spanierman, *Microaggressions in everyday life*. 2020: John Wiley & Sons.

36. Williams, D.R., Race, socioeconomic status, and health the added effects of racism and discrimination. Annals of the New York Academy of Sciences, 1999. 896(1): p. 173-188.

37. Medical News Today. (2023). Effects of racism: How racism can affect physical and mental health. [online] Available at: https://www.medicalnewstoday.com/articles/effects-of-racism.

38. Kline, R. and D. Lewis, The price of fear: estimating the financial cost of bullying and harassment to the NHS in England. Public money & management, 2019. 39(3): p. 166-174.

39. Thomas, R. *Nearly one in three temporary Black and ethnic NHS workers suffer physical violence, internal report reveals*. Independent, 2024. Available at: https://www.independent.co.uk/news/health/nhs-workers-racism-violence-b2606989.html.

40. Courts&Tribunals, Mr S Famojuro v Boots Management Services Ltd and Mrs E Walker: 3219822/2020 and 3204945/2021, E.T. Decisions, Editor. 2023: Welcome to GOV.UK.

41. Sivathasan, N., South Asian anti-black racism: 'We don't marry black people', A. Network, Editor. 2020: BBC NEWS. Available from: https://www.bbc.co.uk/news/av/newsbeat-53395935.

42. Tulsiani, R. The Colour of Power. 2020 [cited 2024; Available at: https://www.green-park.co.uk/insight-reports/the-colour-of-power/s191468/.

43. Burns, C. and D. Connelly. *What will it take to fix pharmacy's stubbornly unchanged ethnicity pay gap?* [cited 2025 January, 19]; Available at: https://pharmaceutical-journal.com/article/feature/what-will-it-take-to-fix-pharmacys-stubbornly-unchanged-ethnicity-pay-gap.

44. Harper, M., et al., *Why African-American women are at greater risk for pregnancy-related death*. Annals of epidemiology, 2007. **17**(3): p. 180-185.

45. Gardner, S. *Serena Williams describes a near-death experience she had after giving birth to daughter Olympia*. [cited 2025 January, 18]; Available at: https://eu.usatoday.com/story/sports/tennis/2022/04/07/serena-williams-near-death-childbirth-complications/9504616002/.

46. Mackey, K., et al., *Racial and ethnic disparities in COVID-19–related infections, hospitalizations, and deaths: a systematic review*. Annals of Internal Medicine, 2021. **174**(3): p. 362-373.

47. Risk assessment survey for pharmacists launched. Available at: https://www.pharmacy.biz/coronavirus/risk-assessment-survey-for-pharmacists-launched/.

48. Coronavirus: 70% of BAME pharmacists have had no risk assessment - survey. Available at: Coronavirus: 70% of BAME pharmacists have had no risk assessment - survey - BBC News.

49. Second phase of the NHS response to COVID-19. Available at: https://www.england.nhs.uk/coronavirus/wp-content/uploads/sites/52/2020/04/second-phase-of-nhs-response-to-covid-19-letter-to-chief-execs-29-april-2020.pdf.

50. Hoffman, K.M., et al., *Racial bias in pain assessment and treatment recommendations, and false beliefs about biological differences between blacks and whites.* Proceedings of the National Academy of Sciences, 2016. **113**(16): p. 4296-4301.

51. Goyal, M.K., et al., *Racial disparities in pain management of children with appendicitis in emergency departments.* JAMA pediatrics, 2015. **169**(11): p. 996-1002.

52. Halvorsrud, K., et al., *Ethnic inequalities and pathways to care in psychosis in England: a systematic review and meta-analysis.* BMC Medicine, 2018. **16**: p. 1-17.

53. Bignall, T., et al., *Racial disparities in mental health.* Race Equality Foundation, 2019.

54. Blumberg, S.J., T.C. Clarke, and D.L. Blackwell, *Racial and ethnic disparities in men's use of mental health treatments.* 2015.

55. Solanki, J., L. Wood, and S. McPherson, *Experiences of adults from a Black ethnic background detained as inpatients under the Mental Health Act (1983).* Psychiatric Rehabilitation Journal, 2023. **46**(1): p. 14.

56. Oldroyd, J., et al., *Diabetes and ethnic minorities.* Postgraduate medical journal, 2005. **81**(958): p. 486-490.

57. Rodríguez, J.E. and K.M. Campbell, *Racial and ethnic disparities in prevalence and care of patients with type 2 diabetes.* Clinical Diabetes, 2017. **35**(1): p. 66-70.

58. DiabetesUK. *Tackling Inequality Commission Report.* 2023; Available at: https://www.diabetes.org.uk/sites/default/files/2023-11/366_Tackling_Inequality_Commission_Report_DIGITAL%20(1).pdf .

59. Chornokur, G., et al., *Disparities at presentation, diagnosis, treatment, and survival in African American men, affected by prostate cancer.* The Prostate, 2011. **71**(9): p. 985-997.

60. Bolarinwa, O.A. and N. Holt, *Barriers to breast and cervical cancer screening uptake among Black, Asian, and Minority Ethnic women in the United Kingdom: evidence from a mixed-methods systematic review.* BMC Health Services Research, 2023. **23**(1): p. 390.

61. Thompson, B., et al., *Breast cancer disparities among women in underserved communities in the USA.* Current breast cancer reports, 2018. **10**: p. 131-141.

62. Fazeli, S., et al., *Access to Breast Cancer Screening: Disparities and Determinants—AJR Expert Panel Narrative Review.* American Journal of Roentgenology, 2024.

63. Li, C.I., K.E. Malone, and J.R. Daling, *Differences in breast cancer stage, treatment, and survival by race and ethnicity.* Archives of internal medicine, 2003. **163**(1): p. 49-56.

64. Miranda, P.Y., W. Tarraf, and H.M. González, *Breast cancer screening and ethnicity in the United States: implications for health disparities research.* Breast cancer research and treatment, 2011. **128**: p. 535-542.

65. Haywood Jr, C. et al., *The impact of race and disease on sickle cell patient wait times in the emergency department.* The American Journal of Emergency Medicine, 2013. **31**(4): p. 651-656.

66. Pulte, D., et al., *Comparison of emergency department wait times in adults with sickle cell disease versus other painful etiologies.* Hemoglobin, 2016. **40**(5): p. 330-334.

67. Kmietowicz, Z., *Patients with sickle cell disease are let down by lack of coordinated NHS care, report finds.* 2023, British Medical Journal Publishing Group.

68. Mahase, E., *Sickle cell disease: inquiry finds serious care failings and racism towards patients.* 2021, British Medical Journal Publishing Group.

69. Willis, A. *Man, 34, dies in London hospital waiting room 2 hours after staff ignore accurate self-diagnosis.* 2024 [cited 2025 January, 19]; Available at: https://www.mylondon.news/news/health/man-34-dies-london-hospital-29895883.

70. Fakoya, I., et al., *HIV testing and sexual health among black African men and women in London, United Kingdom.* JAMA network open, 2019. **2**(3): p. e190864-e190864.

71. DiabetesUK. *Ethnicity and type 2 diabetes.* [cited 2025 January, 19]; Available from: https://www.diabetes.org.uk/about-diabetes/type-2-diabetes/diabetes-ethnicity.

72. CPPE. *Cultural competence hub.* [cited 2025 January, 18]; Available at: https://www.cppe.ac.uk/services/cultural-competence.

73. PDABAME *PDA Anti-Racist Pharmacy Toolkit.* 2022. Available from: https://www.the-pda.org/wp-content/uploads/Anti-racist-Toolkit-FINAL.pdf'.

74. GMC, *Equality, diversity and inclusion Targets, progress and priorities for 2024.*; Available at: https://www.gmc-uk.org/-/media/documents/equality-diversity-and-inclusion---targets-progress-and-priorities-for-2024_pdf-108776261.pdf.

75. .GPhC. *Delivering equality, improving diversity and fostering inclusion. Our strategy for change 2021–26.* 2021 [cited 2025 January, 19]; Available at: https://assets.pharmacyregulation.org/files/document/gphc-equality-diversity-inclusion-strategy-november-2021.pdf.

76. .GPhC. *Racism in pharmacy: report on the roundtable event* 2022 [cited 2025 January, 19]; Available at: https://assets.pharmacyregulation.org/files/document/racism-in-pharmacy-short-report-roundtable_event-november-2022-.pdf.

77. PSA. *General Pharmaceutical Council (GPhC) Performance Review – The monitoring year 2023/24* September 2024; Available at: https://www.professionalstandards.org.uk/sites/default/files/attachments/Monitoring%20report%20GPhC%202023-24.pdf.

78. Clews, G. *Asian and black pharmacists overrepresented in fitness-to-practise concerns, GPhC finds.* 2023 [cited 2025 January, 18]; Available at: https://pharmaceutical-journal.com/article/news/asian-and-black-pharmacists-overrepresented-in-fitness-to-practise-concerns-gphc-finds.

79. Walsh, A., *Judge orders 'incompetent' GPhC to reopen export fraud allegations.* 2024, Communications International Group: Pharmacy Magazine.

80. Khan, G. *Written Medicine.* 2012 [cited 2025 19/01/2025]; Available at: https://writtenmedicine.com/.

81. Norris, D., *Is racism really a problem in our profession?* The Pharmaceutical Journal, 2020. **305**(7942).